CW00420886

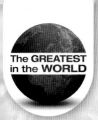
The GREATEST
in the WORLD

illustrated by
Tracy Staskevich

Wendy Green

The Greatest
Slimming &
Healthy Living
Tips in the World

A 'The Greatest in the World' book

www.thegreatestintheworld.com

Illustrations:
Tracy Staskevich
www.tracystaskevich.co.uk

Cover & layout design:
the designcouch
www.designcouch.co.uk

Cover images:
© Liv Friis-Larsen; © Tomo Jesejicnik; © Nikola Hristovski;
© Waugi all courtesy of www.fotolia.com

Copy editor:
Bronwyn Robertson
www.theartsva.com

Series creator/editor:
Steve Brookes

Published in 2008 by
The Greatest in the World Ltd., PO Box 3182
Stratford-upon-Avon, Warwickshire CV37 7XW

A CIP catalogue record for this book is available from the British Library
ISBN 978-1-905151-31-8

Printed and bound in China by 1010 Printing International Ltd.

First, I would like to dedicate this book
to my husband Gordon and to thank him
for his love and total support.

Next, to my late parents.
To my dad, Norman Hughes, for believing in my abilities,
and encouraging me to return to writing, and my mam,
Doreen, for instilling in me a love of books.

Last, but by no means least, I'd like to mention my son
Paul, my daughter Kathryn and my two grandsons Scott
and Dylan, all of whom I'm extremely proud!

A few words from Wendy …

In the UK there are more commercial diets and diet books to choose from than ever before, and each year thousands of people join a gym – yet nearly one in two men and one in three women is overweight. The nation as a whole is far heavier than it was fifty years ago. The reasons are simple – we eat more fatty, refined and sugary foods than our parents and grandparents did, and we aren't as physically active in our daily lives.

I've been interested in health and staying slim since I was a teenager. When I gained weight during my teens and early twenties, I lost it by dieting. During my mid-thirties, the pounds crept on again. I did nothing about it, until my late thirties, when I was studying nutrition as part of a health degree. This time I applied what I'd learned and ate a more balanced diet. I also realised my weight gain was linked to eating for reasons other than hunger, so I worked on having a more normal relationship with food. This time the weight came off, and has stayed off.

I firmly believe staying slim, healthy and fit, involves finding a balanced way of eating and living that suits you in the long-term, rather than following a strict diet – a short-term solution that will inevitably fail. It's also about building more activity into your daily life, rather than joining a gym you're unlikely to attend. In this book you'll find tips based on my personal experiences and what I've learned from studying nutrition and health for a number of years.

Contents

Dieting is
wishful shrinking.

Anon

Think thin

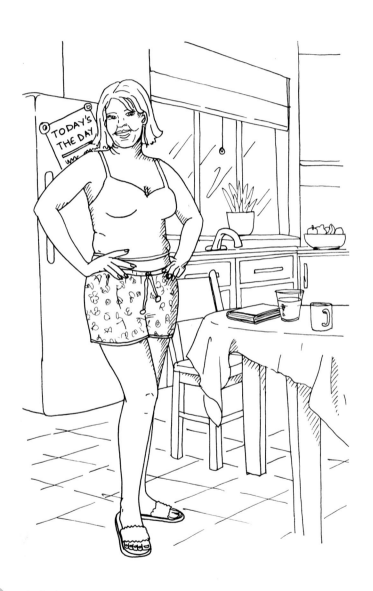

chapter 1
Think thin

We're constantly bombarded with information about healthy eating. There are more commercial diets to choose from than ever before. Yet nearly a quarter of adults in the UK are obese. Clearly, knowing what and how much we should eat in order to be a healthy weight is only part of the story; what and why we eat is also strongly linked to unconscious emotions and past experiences. Many of us indulge in emotional, or comfort, eating to help us deal with negative emotions such as fear, anger, sadness, and low self-esteem. Often we turn to foods we learned to associate with comfort during childhood, such as chocolate, crisps, and ice cream. This chapter looks at the psychological aspects of weight gain and weight loss, and how to harness the power of your subconscious mind to help you lose weight.

No more excuses!

Go on, be honest! Do you find excuses for being overweight, such as "I don't really eat much, it's my metabolism" or "I've always been big"? If you're overweight, research shows that you're likely to have a faster metabolism than a slimmer person, because you need more calories to maintain your weight and body's basic functioning. And even if you have always been overweight, you can still lose weight by changing your eating habits and activity levels.

It's in my genes!

"Other members of my family are big" is another common excuse. Whilst research suggests 1 in 6 people in the UK carries the FTO or so-called 'fat' gene that can make them 3kg (7lbs) heavier than those who don't, this needs to be put into context. Only 30% of those with one flawed FTO gene and 70% of those with 2, are more likely to be overweight. Almost 1 in 4 people in the UK are obese. A person carrying this amount of excess weight isn't classified as obese. So the majority of people with a weight problem can't blame it on their genes!

What you're more likely to have inherited from your family members are the lifestyle habits that lead to weight gain, such as eating a poor diet, overeating, and being inactive.

Generally, unless you're suffering from a medical condition, or taking a drug linked with weight gain, if you're overweight you're taking in more calories than you're burning off. It's that simple.

Quick tip

HUNGER PANGS

Another common excuse for not losing weight is "I'm always hungry". The answer to this is – you don't have to go hungry to lose weight. If you eat healthy, balanced meals, you're less likely to feel hungry in between meals. But if you do experience hunger pangs, choose sensible snacks, such as those suggested further on in the book. Facing up to the real reasons why you're overweight, could be your first step doing something about it.

Are you ready to slim?

You'll only change your eating habits when you're ready. That might sound obvious, but it's surprising how many people state they really should lose weight, but do nothing about it. Research suggests this is because most people go through a cycle of stages before they make permanent behaviour changes, and will only be successful if they progress to the stage where they're ready to commit to making the necessary changes.

Psychologists Prochaska and DiClemente identified six stages in the cycle: Pre-contemplation, Contemplation, Preparation, Action, Maintenance, and Relapse.

Pre-contemplation – This is the stage where you are either unaware of the need to lose weight, or simply have no desire to lose weight.

Contemplation – At this stage you are becoming aware of the need or desire to change your habits and are seriously thinking about doing so. You are likely to have a reason for this change of attitude. Perhaps you're concerned about your health, or maybe you want to improve your appearance. You might start looking at what is required in order to lose weight, i.e. lifestyle changes, in terms of what and how much you eat and how much exercise you take. But you're not quite ready to make these changes.

Preparation – You've decided to take action. You're beginning to make serious plans to help you achieve your goal, such as identifying your target weight, the date by which you want to reach it, and how you intend to achieve it.

Action – This is the point where you are ready to take active steps to change your lifestyle. You will now start making the changes necessary to bring about weight loss. Your level of motivation is likely to be high and you find it easy to stick to your new eating and activity habits.

Maintenance – This is the hardest part of changing your lifestyle, because the initial enthusiasm might have worn off. Perhaps people are no longer complimenting you on your new shape. Old patterns of comfort eating and overindulging in the wrong types of foods seem tempting. This is the time when you might need support and encouragement from family and friends. It might help if you revisit the reasons why you wanted to lose weight in the first place and remind yourself of your achievements. Identify situations where you're tempted to overeat and plan strategies to help you resist. Reward yourself with non-food items such as a new perfume, or new clothes.

Relapse – You've returned to your old habits! The key to dealing with this stage is not to panic. Accept that it happens to most people. Then return to the contemplation stage and begin the cycle again. Evidence suggests many people go through the process of change 3 or more times before finally leaving behind the lifestyle that made them overweight. The important point to remember is that becoming slimmer and healthier isn't about sticking to a rigid diet. It's more about making lifestyle changes on a long-term basis. If you occasionally overeat it shouldn't lead to weight gain, providing you stick to healthy habits most of the time.

Where are you in the cycle?

If you haven't started trying to lose weight, but you're obviously thinking about it, because you're reading this book, then you're at the contemplation stage. The next step for you is preparation. This is a good time to keep a food diary to identify your eating patterns. You could then make an action plan, setting out your goal and the steps you need to take to achieve it, perhaps incorporating some of the weight loss tips outlined in this book that appeal to you. Then take action by following your action plan.

If you've lost weight in the past and then regained it, you're at the relapse stage. It's important that you don't give up, but find ways that suit you to eat less and be more active. This book offers you lots of ideas on how to do this.

What's your motivation?

Losing weight can be difficult, especially initially. So when you're finding it tough to stick to your new eating habits, identifying why you want to slim and focussing on the rewards, can help you to stay on the straight and narrow. For example, your motivation might be that you want to slip into that little black dress, or you want to look good on the beach, or that you simply want to feel better.

Focusing regularly on the long-term pleasure you'll gain from achieving your weight loss goal can help you to resist the short-term pleasures of overeating.

Great expectations!

Some people hold the mistaken belief that if they lose weight, their lives will be perfect. They attach all kinds of attributes to slimness, such as confidence, success, and attractiveness. Consequently they fear being slim. What if they don't live up to their own or other's expectations? Being overweight becomes a way of avoiding having to be this perfect person with a perfect life.

For others, the opposite might be true – they lose weight because of their belief that their lives will be perfect once they become slim. But, once they lose weight, they realise this isn't the case. Disillusioned, many then start to comfort eat and consequently regain the weight they lost, and more.

Weight loss might improve your health and boost confidence, but you will still be the same person, with your own unique personality and traits. Changing your shape will not magically change your life, it will simply change your shape!

Once you've accepted this fact, you might find it easier to lose excess weight, because you'll no longer have unrealistic expectations of yourself, and what your life will be like once you become thin.

Self-talk and size

Self-talk is a term used to describe the ongoing conversation we have with ourselves. If your self-talk is negative as in "I'll never lose weight. I'm fat and I can't change" it'll perpetuate a negative self-image which your actions will reflect, probably in the form of overeating. Equally, if you make sure your self-talk is constructive, by creating positive affirmations using the methods outlined below, you will find yourself acting in ways that support this positive view of yourself.

Affirm and slim

An affirmation is a positive statement you make about yourself. It needs to be personal, so use the word 'I'. It must be positive, so state what you want to achieve, not what you don't. It's also more effective if you write it as though it's happening now. So a good weight loss affirmation would incorporate all of these points. For example "I am slim and healthy" rather than "I will not be overweight and unfit". This imprints in your subconscious mind a clear image of the result you want to achieve, as though you've already achieved it, e.g. "I am slim, healthy, happy, and energetic". Attaching positive emotions to your goal will make it seem more real and achievable. You'll also see results more quickly.

To fix your affirmation in your subconscious mind, first read it. Next, shut your eyes and see the picture your words conjure up. Picture yourself experiencing your goal in detail. Visualise yourself slim. Imagine the clothes you'll wear. Feel the emotions you've attached to your goal. Hear the words your family and friends will use to compliment you on your appearance. Reading, picturing, feeling, and hearing your affirmation has a powerful effect on your subconsious mind. Do this on a daily basis and you should quickly find yourself adopting behaviours to support this new image you have of yourself, i.e. healthy habits, such as eating a balanced diet and being more active.

Seeing is believing

Remember, your subconscious mind can't tell the difference between what's happened in reality, and what's occurred in your imagination. If you regularly visualise yourself slim, your subconscious mind will believe you're already slim and you'll find yourself acting like a slim person.

Set specific and realistic targets

Set yourself a specific and realistic target such as "I will lose 450g (1lb) per week". You're more likely to be successful than if you simply state "I want to lose weight", or if you set yourself unrealistic goals such as "I will lose 6.5kg (1 stone) in a month".

Identify your eating patterns

Keep a food and drink diary for a week, recording not only when you ate, but also how hungry you were, what and how much you ate, where, who with, and how you felt at the time, e.g. stressed, happy, sad, angry, upset. This will help you identify the eating patterns that are sabotaging your efforts to lose weight. For example, eating when you're stressed or bored rather than hungry. You can then plan strategies to overcome them.

Sample Food Diary

Date/ Time	Hunger level	Food Eaten /Drinks	Where & who with	Feelings

Mind mindless eating

It's important that you record everything you eat. If you habitually eat the kids' or your partner's leftovers without thinking, you need to include it in your diary. If you regularly taste-test while you cook – that counts too! Eating just 100 calories a day more than you need can lead to a 4.5kg (10lb) weight gain in a year. Make it a rule to throw away your family's leftovers and stop taste-testing in the kitchen; this could help you lose pounds!

Manage stress

Research shows that long-term stress leads to over-production of the stress hormones, adrenaline and cortisol. Eating sugary and fatty foods seems to counteract their effects by inducing feelings of calm. If you tend to overeat or binge on junk foods when stressed, try to find other ways to relax. For example, practise deep breathing, exercise, listen to music, or drink chamomile tea. After a stressful day at work, enjoy a long relaxing soak in the bath, rather than heading straight for the food cupboard. Do whatever works for you. If you're stressed because of a problem, try to find a solution, or talk it through with someone you trust, rather than turning to food.

Beat boredom

If you tend to eat when bored, plan ways to beat boredom that don't involve food. Read that new novel you've been meaning to read. Catch up with the friend you haven't seen for ages. Find a new interest that excites you. That way you'll 'eat to live' rather than 'live to eat'.

Feel rather than 'eat' emotions

If you comfort eat to suppress emotions such as anger or hurt, explore ways to express and deal with your feelings, such as talking them through with an appropriate person, or writing them down. Identify any underlying issues or problems and seek solutions, so that you can treat food as fuel for your body, rather than an escape from your emotions. Food might provide a temporary distraction or comfort, but the emotions or problems you're trying to distance yourself from will still be there, probably with the added problem of weight gain.

So next time you find yourself dipping into the biscuit tin ask yourself "Am I hungry for food, or is something bothering me?"

Swap bad habits for good ones

A habit is something you do several times until it becomes ingrained in your patterns of behaviour and you can do it almost without thinking. What you eat, and how often, is largely based on habits – often formed during childhood. So to lose weight you need to replace bad eating habits with good ones. Once you have carried out the new behaviour several times, it too becomes a habit and therefore easier to stick to.

Quick tip

FOLLOW THE 80:20 RULE
Don't beat yourself up if you overindulge sometimes. Evidence suggests that if you eat healthily 80% of the time, you needn't worry about the other 20%.

Meal planner

Planning your meals in advance makes it less likely that you'll grab a takeaway, or fill up on junk food. Take healthy snacks to work with you such as nuts, seeds, fruit, or chopped raw vegetables, so that you're less likely to be tempted by the biscuit tin. Make your own packed lunch, or find a sandwich shop that offers wholemeal bread and healthy fillings. If you must eat fast food, think before you order about how you can make it healthier.

To weigh, or not to weigh?

Stepping onto the scales boosts morale – if you've lost weight. If you haven't, it can depress and demotivate – especially if you've eaten healthily and been more active. Take a long-term view – if your weight is generally going down, the occasional hiccup doesn't matter.

Regular weighing can help weight loss and maintenance by acting as an early warning system – a few pounds are easier to shift than a stone or more! But for some vulnerable people, especially teenage girls, weighing too often can result in an unhealthy obsession with weight.

So weigh yourself as often as you feel comfortable. Every few days is fine, but note your weight can fluctuate by several pounds, for reasons such as hormonal fluctuations in women, water retention and changes in muscle mass. Strength training can increase weight, because muscle weighs more than fat. Here, it's better to monitor your progress with a tape measure, or how your clothes fit.

Enough is as
good as a feast.

Anon

Eat less

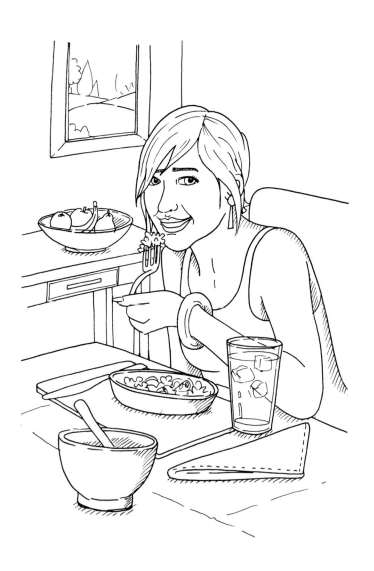

chapter 2
Eat less

To lose weight we need to take in fewer calories than we burn off. The best way to do this is to eat a healthy, balanced diet on a long-term basis, rather than following fad diets on a short-term basis. Such diets tend to deprive you of your favourite foods, making you more likely to want to eat them and eventually give in to your cravings. However, it's still possible to gain weight eating healthy food – if you eat more than your body needs. So this section suggests dietary and behavioural changes to help you cut down on the amount of food you eat, without having to count calories or stick to a strict diet regime.

Eating less can be difficult. We live in an environment where food, particularly fast and convenience food, is available 24 hours a day. It's easier than ever to eat too much generally, but particularly food high in fat and sugar and low in nutritional value. Whenever we feel the urge to eat, it's very easy to do so. To help you beat this, I've included ideas to make overeating more difficult.

Introduce new behaviours gradually, perhaps only one at a time. Even if you only adopt one change, it could be enough to change your eating habits for life and enable you to lose weight and keep it off permanently. Remember, small changes can make a big difference when it comes to weight management - even cutting out one biscuit each day could lead to a loss of 4.5kg (10 lbs) in weight in a year!

Body Mass Indicator

Before you make any changes to your eating habits, check whether you're overweight. The current most popular method is to work out your Body Mass Indicator (BMI).

To calculate your BMI (which is always calculated in metric), multiply your height in metres by your height in metres. Then divide your weight in kilograms by this figure.

For example, if you were 1.6m tall and weighed 65kg you would work it out like this:

1.6 metres x 1.6 metres = 2.56

BMI = 65 divided by 2.56 = 25.39

BMI Ratings

Less than 18.5 – underweight

18.5 – 24.9 – healthy weight

25.0 – 29.9 – overweight

30.0 – 39.9 – obese

40.0 and above – morbid obesity

A BMI of 25.39 would indicate the need to lose a little weight. But remember your BMI is only a guide. A muscular person with little fat would still have a high BMI, as it measures weight, rather than fat, in relation to height.

BE WAIST WISE

Another indicator that you need to lose weight is your waist size. Carrying too much fat around your middle increases your risk of serious health problems such as heart disease, high blood pressure, and diabetes. A waist size of 80cm (32 inches) for a woman and 94cm (37 inches) for a man, indicates increased risk. For women, an 88cm (35 inch) or above, and for men a 102cm (40 inches), or above, waist means you're at high risk of ill-health. To reduce your waist size you need to combine healthy eating with being more active.

Pills that can plump

There are numerous common medicines for conditions such as hayfever, asthma, depression, travel sickness, colds, and insomnia, which can lead to weight gain due to increased appetite or fluid retention. Antihistamines, steroids, antidepressants, and the contraceptive pill, are just some of the medications that could make weight loss more difficult. If you're taking a medication regularly and struggling with losing weight, a discussion with your GP or pharmacist is a good idea. They might be able to offer an alternative medication that will have less effect on your weight. It's probably even more important that you follow the advice on healthy eating and activity, not only to avoid weight gain, but to improve your health generally.

Chop or change!

Keep a food diary as outlined in the *Think Thin* section. Check what and how much you're eating. Most people underestimate how much they actually eat and find this exercise an eye-opener. Then decide what you could cut down on, or omit altogether – for example one biscuit instead of two, no cream in your coffee, no mid-afternoon snack.

Look for lower-fat alternatives to your favourite foods, so that you eat less fat. For example oven chips instead of fried; low-fat, rather than creamy yoghurt; twiglets, rather than crisps. For more food swap ideas, go to the Eat Healthier chapter.

Quick tip

CUT 100
Cutting around 100 calories from your daily intake will enable you to lose around 4.5kg (10lb) in a year. That could mean simply cutting out one biscuit a day, or 6 teaspoons of sugar, or 1 packet of crisps. A small change with a big result!

Less is more!

When you reduce your food intake, you will probably find that you enjoy your food far more. When you overeat, you go beyond the point when eating is pleasurable.

Go for low GI …

The Glycaemic Index (GI) indicates the rate a food raises the level of sugar in the blood. Carbohydrates with a high GI include refined foods such as white bread, pastries, sugary drinks, and sweets, which are easily converted into glucose and cause your blood sugar to rise rapidly.

Carbohydrates with a low GI, such as multigrain bread, porridge, sweet potatoes, pasta, and basmati or brown rice, take longer to digest and cause your blood glucose to rise slowly, making you feel full longer and therefore eat less. Low GI foods also reduce the risk of type 2 diabetes.

For a low GI diet, replace all refined carbohydrates such as white bread, biscuits, pastries, and sweets, with whole grains. Eat lots of fruit and vegetables, low fat dairy products, such as yoghurt, skimmed/semi-skimmed milk, and low fat cheese, and small amounts of nuts, fish, and lean meat. Leave the skins on potatoes to keep their Glycaemic Index low – eating potatoes without the skin enables the glucose to be digested more quickly. New potatoes boiled in their skins have the lowest GI.

Sticking to these types of foods also helps to dispel excess fat around the stomach, which is believed to increase the risk of heart disease, high blood pressure, and type 2 diabetes.

…..and high satiety

Satiety is the term used to describe the feeling of fullness and satisfaction you experience after eating. The satiety index has been devised to rate foods in terms of their ability to satisfy hunger. The longer a food makes you feel full, the higher its rating. Research suggests that high-volume, low-calorie foods make you feel content more quickly and for longer, so that you're less likely to overeat. Foods with a high water content, such as fruit, vegetables and fish, fit into this category.

If you eat high-calorie low-volume foods, such as full-fat cheese or chocolate, you're likely to ingest a lot more calories before your brain signals to you that you are full. For example, if you ate grapes in their dried form, as raisins, you would take in 100 calories after eating only one quarter of a cup, but you could eat a cup full of fresh grapes and still only consume 100 calories. So if you want to lose weight, aim at eating foods with lots of bulk, but low in calories. Foods with a high satiety score include baked potatoes, fish, porridge, oranges, apples, grapes, wholewheat pasta, steak, and unsweetened popcorn.

Quick tip

EAT BREAKFAST

Studies show that people who eat breakfast tend to eat less during the day and are therefore usually slimmer. Choose low GI foods such as whole grain bread or porridge. Adding protein in the form of skimmed or semi-skimmed milk, or eggs, will keep your blood sugar steady.

Loaded

Another term you might come across is Glycaemic Load
(GL). It's possible for a food to have a high GI, but a low GL.
Confused? In a nutshell, GL is a measure of how much
a 'normal' portion of a particular food affects blood sugar.
The Glycaemic Index is based on a portion containing 50g
(2oz) of carbohydrate, which could be quite a large amount.
So, it's possible for a high GI food to have a low GL.
For example, ice cream has a high GI, but a low GL – when
you eat just a couple of scoops. Basically, this means you can
eat foods like ice cream in small amounts, without affecting
your blood sugar too much. Again the message is, keep refined
sugary and starchy foods to a minimum!

Protein power

Eating protein foods such as meat, fish, eggs, and cheese at
each meal can help you to eat less, and burn more calories
and fat. Protein makes you feel fuller for longer, because it
slows down the rate that the body digests food. When eaten
with carbohydrates, glucose is released more slowly into the
bloodstream. Research showed that people whose diet was
about one third protein ate, on average, 441 calories less each
day than those whose diet contained around one sixth protein.

Protein also boosts the metabolism for up to 3 hours, so you
burn more calories. It's claimed that the body burns around one
third of the calories from protein whilst processing it. It also
encourages the body to burn fat for energy. But beware, animal
proteins are high in saturated fats, so go for low-fat dairy foods
and lean meats.

Go to work on an egg!

It seems this famous advert slogan, encouraging us to eat eggs, offered good advice. A study showed that women who ate two eggs and toast at breakfast felt so full and satisfied, they ate nearly 300 calories less each day, than women who ate bagels and cream cheese. Another similar study in Rochester backed up these findings. Eggs are a good, cheap source of protein, vitamins A, B2 and D, calcium, and iodine. They used to have a bad press because of their cholesterol content, but it's now generally agreed that saturated fats have more influence on cholesterol levels than cholesterol in food. They're also low in salt. The healthiest way to eat them is either boiled or poached.

Sip soup

Non-creamy soups such as vegetable, carrot and coriander or tomato and basil are nutritious, low in calories and filling. A study showed that eating chicken and vegetable soup keeps you full for an hour longer than if you drink water, then eat chicken and vegetables. It seems soup is more filling because the water and solids combined stay in the stomach longer.

Eat your favourite foods

Basing your diet on foods you really enjoy, rather than simply on foods you feel you should eat, means you're less likely to feel deprived and go on an eating binge. It's human nature to want what you think you can't have! However, you might need to adapt your favourite recipes to make them lower in fat and sugar. Aim at developing a taste for healthier foods, so that you can still satisfy your palate, whilst managing your weight.

Chew gum

Chewing gum between meals has been shown to reduce appetite and decrease food intake at mealtimes by around a third. Choose sugar-free for fewer calories and better dental health.

Quick tip

DON'T SHOP ON AN EMPTY STOMACH!
Eat before you go food shopping. Studies show that when you shop on an empty stomach you're more likely to buy fatty, sugary foods.

Shopping list

Writing a shopping list before you go, and sticking to it, also helps to ensure you buy only the foods you really need. Set yourself a time limit – the less time you spend at the supermarket the less likely you are to buy things that aren't on your list.

Small is beautiful

Research reveals that people eat up to 45% more food when it's in a large pack. In one study, people with a large box containing 400g (1lb) of spaghetti ate up to a third more than another group, who were given a small box containing the same amount of spaghetti. So go for foods in smaller packs at the supermarket.

Self-checkout

Evidence suggests that using the self-checkout till makes you 50% less likely to buy foods on impulse.

MAKE MEALTIMES AN OCCASION
Sit at the table. Set the table properly and add little touches like napkins or flowers to make it look inviting. Play relaxing music. If you make meal times more of an occasion you'll be less likely to bolt your food and overeat.

Make snacking an occasion too

If you make it a rule to eat snacks from a plate at the table too, you'll be less likely to snack on impulse, because it'll require more effort than simply grabbing food and eating it.

Drink more water

Drink more water – it'll fill you up and prevent you mistaking thirst for hunger.

Don't eat ….

- Because it's a meal time.
- Because you're starting a diet tomorrow.
- Because other people are eating.
- Because something is 'eating' you.
- Because you've worked hard and you deserve it.

Eat ….

Only when you're hungry, and stop when you're full. When you eat only in response to stomach (physiological) hunger, rather than mouth (psychological) hunger, you're eating in keeping with your body's needs, rather than your emotional ones. If you're normally an emotional eater, this means you'll be eating less.

Recognise real hunger

Recognise how your body signals when it's hungry. For most people, hunger manifests itself with contractions in the stomach, but some feel it in the chest or throat. You might experience similar feelings when your appetite is stimulated by the thought, sight, or smell of food. However these sensations are usually temporary, whereas real hunger doesn't fade. Generally, if you have to ask yourself "Am I hungry?" you're probably not!

Rate your hunger

Reduce the likelihood of overeating by rating your hunger before you eat. Try measuring your hunger on a scale of 1 to 4, with 1 signifying you're full, 2 signifying you're peckish, 3 signifying you're hungry and 4 signifying you're ravenous. This will help you to determine how much food you need. For example, if you rate your hunger as a 2, perhaps a smaller plate of food, or a snack, rather than a full meal, will do. If you wait until your hunger rating is 4, you're more likely to crave sweet, starchy foods to give your lowered blood sugar an instant boost, so try to eat when your rating is no more than 3.

Hungry for what?

Your appetite is there not just to tell you when you're hungry, but also what kind of food your body needs – if you listen to it. Your individual nutritional requirements are dependent on many things, including your age, gender, and activity levels. For instance, if you've been physically active all day, you're likely to crave more starchy, energy-producing foods, than if you'd just sat in a chair. If you eat what your body is hungry for, you'll probably find you'll be satisfied with less food than if you just eat whatever is to hand.

Heat up

Turn down the air-conditioning at the office and at home, during hot weather and you should find your appetite decreases.

Quick tip

FEMALES NEED LESS FOOD
If you're a woman, remember that in general women need around 500 calories fewer than men, so make sure you serve yourself smaller portions – about a fifth less than your partner's.

Chew it over

An American study showed that people who chew their food well tend to eat around 70 calories less at each meal and still feel full an hour later.

Portion control

To maintain a healthy weight, it's vital that you control your portion sizes. Even if you eat healthy foods, if you eat too much of them you'll gain weight.

An easy guide :

- Carbohydrate foods such as pasta and rice: 2 handfuls.
- Vegetables/salad: 2 handfuls.
- Protein foods such as meat, cheese, eggs and fish: 1 handful.
- Nuts: 1 small handful.
- Fats and oils: 15ml (1 tablespoon) or less.

Use a smaller plate

Evidence suggests that the bigger the portion size, the more people will eat; the 'supersizing' of fast food meals is one of the factors blamed for the rise in obesity. Eating from a smaller plate automatically cuts your portion sizes.

Slow down!

If you eat quickly, you can end up eating a lot more food than you need before your brain realises. So try to eat slowly and focus on each mouthful. Savour the smell, texture, and taste of your food. You'll enjoy it more and find it easier to recognise when you've eaten enough, because your body will have time to release leptin, the hormone that signals satisfaction. You'll probably notice that your enjoyment of your food declines as you fill up. This is your body's way of signalling that you've eaten enough. Aim to stop eating when this happens.

Conscious eating

When you're tempted to overeat, stop and ask yourself "Do I really want this food, or am I just eating it because it's there?". Then make a choice whether or not to eat some, or all, of the food. This puts you in control, rather than the food.

Avoid distractions

Don't watch TV or read whilst you're eating. By avoiding distractions and giving your food your full attention, you'll probably find that you eat less.

Tune in to your taste buds

When you start eating, focus on the flavour of your food. Does it taste good? It's easy to eat a plateful of food without really tasting it. When you take the time to taste what you're eating, you might decide it's not all that nice and choose not to eat it.

Avoid 'empty plate syndrome'

As a child you might have been encouraged to clear your plate and told it was wasteful not to. Remember, your hunger should determine how much you eat, not the portion size. Practise leaving food on your plate until you feel comfortable with it. If it makes you feel any better, feed your leftovers to the birds!

Take a break

It can take 15 to 20 minutes for your brain to register that your stomach is full. So if you pause for a few minutes before reaching for that second helping or dessert, you might find you're no longer hungry and can do without.

Beat buffet binging

It's easy to overeat at buffets — many people ignore their body's 'full-up' signals and overeat when faced with a vast array of foods. This is because when we eat only one or two foods, we soon become tired of the taste. If we select lots of different foods and tastes, our taste buds are stimulated each time and we're more likely to overeat. Try the following strategies to beat buffet binging:

- Visit the buffet table only once. Avoid too much pastry. Fill your plate with mainly protein foods such as chicken—minus the skin—other lean meats, carbohydrate, such as bread or rice, and plenty of salad.
- If you eat dessert, make it a small portion.
- Be selective. Only choose foods you enjoy.
- Eat slowly and focus on your food as well as the conversation.
- Talking is a good ploy to prevent you eating too quickly!
- Overindulging in alcohol can lead to overeating, because it stimulates the appetite and weakens resolve, so alternate alcoholic drinks with non-alcoholic ones.

Learn to say 'no'

When you're a guest at someone's home, or attending a function, don't allow yourself to be pressured into eating food out of politeness. When you feel you've eaten enough, or when you're just not hungry, don't be afraid to compliment your host on their delicious food, but state firmly that you just can't eat any more, or you're not hungry.

Eat less in company

Research shows that people eat around a third more food when they eat with another person, as opposed to eating alone. Eat with 3 and you're likely to eat three quarters more. Eat with a group of 7 or more people and you could eat up to 90% more. If you're eating at home you're likely to continue eating until everyone has finished, thus possibly eating more than you need to. When eating out we tend to want to prolong the whole eating and social experience, so we're more likely to order a dessert, even if we're full.

To counteract the tendency to eat more in company, aim to be the last person to start eating and the slowest eater. Engaging in conversation is a good ploy – it's difficult to talk and eat at the same time!

Do something different

There's evidence that changing your routine by doing something different every day can lead to weight loss. In a study, people following this advice lost an average of nearly 1.5kg (3lbs) a month, without consciously changing their eating or exercise habits. It seems this works because doing new and interesting things forces you to break the old habits which have prevented you from losing weight. One woman found that by breaking her routine of sitting in front of the TV each night, she started to do things she'd been putting off doing, such as clearing the clutter in her home. She went on to take up new interests, and as a side effect she lost weight. It appears that as people gain more fulfilment in their lives, their weight decreases.

You're also less likely to focus on food and eat just for the sake of it. One woman described herself as being less interested in food and more interested in achieving more in her life.

So, if you've thought about trying salsa dancing or rock climbing, or even just listening to another radio station or reading a different newspaper, give it a go – you've nothing to lose but excess weight!

Clean your teeth

Try cleaning your teeth after your evening meal. The fresh, minty taste should make you feel less inclined to snack on sweet foods afterwards.

Sleep and slim

Too little sleep has been shown to affect hormones and metabolism, making overeating and weight gain more likely. A recent study showed that people who don't get enough sleep eat nearly half as much more than those who do. A hormone called leptin regulates how much we eat by giving the signal of fullness when we've eaten enough. Ghrelin is a hormone that increases hunger –especially for high carbohydrate foods.

People who sleep poorly have been found to have lower levels of leptin and higher levels of ghrelin, and as a result are more likely to overeat. If you feel that lack of sleep might be contributing to your weight problem, start taking steps now to ensure you get more sleep and you could find yourself eating less and losing weight. Even an extra twenty minutes has been shown to lead to weight loss.

Food is an
important part
of a balanced diet.

Fran Lebowitz

Eat healthily

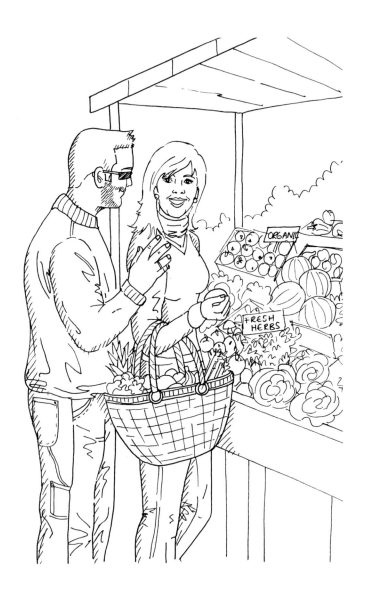

chapter 3
Eat healthily

Being overweight is a risk factor for several health problems. These include high blood pressure, coronary heart disease, stroke, some cancers, type 2 diabetes, osteoarthritis, liver disease and fertility problems. Experts warn that unless obesity rates are reduced, many will die up to nine years earlier than they need to, or have an old age blighted by poor health.

So it's generally accepted that if you want to live a long and healthy life, you need to maintain a healthy weight. If you want to lose weight, it's best to avoid fad diets. Many such diets, including some of the commercial ones, are nutritionally unbalanced and, in the long-term, lead to weight gain. This is mainly because many of them are so restrictive, it's impossible to stick to them for any length of time. They may result in weight loss, but as soon as the dieter reverts to 'normal' eating, weight is regained. Often the dieter ends up heavier, because a low-calorie diet will encourage the body to go into 'starvation mode', which means that the metabolism slows down. The body then needs fewer calories, so when more are consumed, they're stored as fat.

Yo-yo dieting, where a person loses weight, regains it and then goes on to lose it again, has been shown to endanger health, because it damages vital organs such as the heart, liver and kidneys and raises the risk of stroke, diabetes and heart disease.

It may sound boring, but the secret of healthy, long-lasting weight management is a healthy, balanced diet, along with regular physical activity. Not only is this more effective, it's also cheaper – the cost of attending commercial diet classes can often mean that the only pounds you lose are the ones in your purse or wallet!

The current guidelines for a balanced diet suggest that around a third of the diet should consist of carbohydrates such as bread, cereal and potatoes and that these should be wholegrain where possible. Fruit and vegetables should make up another third of your diet. The remaining third should be shared roughly equally between dairy and protein foods and a slightly smaller amount of fatty, sugary foods. Healthy eating is really just about getting the balance right. You can still eat fatty and sugary foods – so long as you view them as a treat and eat them sparingly. Eating too many refined and sugary foods has been linked to raised blood sugar levels, which can lead to diabetes, obesity, high blood pressure, heart disease and stroke. But when only your favourite high-calorie treat will do – indulge in a small amount. This is better than trying to stick to an impossibly strict diet, whilst craving a food you're not 'allowed'. Eventually you're likely to give in to the craving and go on an eating 'binge', or just abandon the diet. Following a balanced diet helps you to have a more normal relationship with food, rather than an all or nothing 'diet, or no-diet' approach.

This section offers suggestions to help you follow these guidelines, control your weight and dramatically improve your health, without having to stick to a restrictive diet, or spend a fortune on special foods.

PERFECT PLATE

For an easy way to ensure a balanced meal, fill roughly one third of your plate with vegetables and/or fruit, a third with carbohydrates and add a handful of a high-protein food.

Feeling fruity?

Eating more fruit and vegetables is probably the easiest way to improve your long-term health and lose weight. Fruit and vegetables generally contain various vitamins, minerals, and phytochemicals (plant chemicals), which offer numerous benefits to health. Studies have shown that people who lose weight tend to keep it off if they base their meals around fruit and vegetables, probably because these foods provide a feeling of fullness, leaving less room for sugary, fatty foods. Current recommendations are that we should eat at least five portions of fruit and veg a day.

Eat a rainbow

To benefit from a wide range of phytonutrients, make sure you eat fruit and vegetables across the spectrum of colours. These pigments indicate the compounds contained in the plant. Each compound offers various disease- preventing properties. The red of tomatoes comes from lycopene. Anthocyanins give fruits such as strawberries, cherries, blueberries, plums, and grapes their red, blue or purple hues. The orange pigment in carrots is beta-carotene. Read more about them in the *Superfoods, herbs & spices* chapter.

What's a portion?

All fruit and vegetables, including fresh, frozen, canned, dried, and pure juices, count. But no matter how much juice you drink, it only counts as one portion, because it doesn't contain all of the fibre of the whole fruit. Also, the sugars are more concentrated and can cause damage to teeth. Potatoes, sweet potatoes, and yams are starchy and are classed as carbohydrates, rather than vegetables. Pulses such as beans, lentils, and peas only count as one portion, whatever amount you eat, because like potatoes, they're quite starchy and don't contain all of the vitamins and antioxidants that fruit and vegetables do.

The World Health Organisation recommends that we eat at least 400g (1lb) of fruit and vegetables daily to obtain the nutrients we need for good health. It was decided that the easiest way to achieve this was by eating at least 5 x 80g (2½oz) portions daily. This translates roughly into:

- One piece of medium-sized fruit such as an apple, banana, orange, pear, or peach.
- A slice of large fruit, for example melon, mango, or pineapple.
- A cupful of grapes, cherries, or berries such as strawberries or raspberries.
- Two kiwis, plums, or satsumas.
- Half a grapefruit or avocado.
- 15ml (1 tablespoon) of dried fruit, such as raisins or sultanas.
- Three dried apricots.

- A glass (roughly 100ml/3½fl.oz) of fruit or vegetable juice.
- A small can (roughly 200g/7½oz) of fruit, preferably in natural juice.
- A dessert bowl of salad.
- Roughly 100g (4oz) of vegetables, such as frozen or mushy peas, boiled carrots, or broccoli.
- 100g (4oz) of pulses such as baked beans, kidney beans, peas, or lentils.
- The vegetables included in meals like a vegetable curry, lasagne, stir-fry, or casserole.

Salad days

Salads are a great way to make sure you eat the recommended 5 fruit and vegetables per day. However choose your dressing carefully. Full-fat mayonnaises, salad creams, and dressings will add extra calories. Go for balsamic vinegar, or swap full-fat dressings for a low-fat version. Or mix ordinary salad cream or mayonnaise with an equal amount of low-fat yogurt for a lower-fat version.

Organic vs non-organic

A growing body of research points to organic fruit and vegetables providing more nutrients than conventionally grown crops. So if you can afford it, opt for organic.

However, non-organic produce is OK so long as you wash or peel it before eating, to reduce any risk from pesticides. For more information on organic produce and details of suppliers, visit **www.whyorganic.org**.

Take five

Find it hard to get your five portions of fruit and vegetables every day? Here are some suggestions:

- Drink fruit juice at breakfast.

- Add a sliced apple, or banana, or a few strawberries to your breakfast cereal.

- Carry a small packet of dried fruit such as raisins, or dried apricots in your bag.

- Add salad to sandwiches at lunch time.

- Snack on fruit or raw vegetables such as carrots, celery, or peppers. Take some to work. Put them on your desk so you're more likely to eat them.

- Add grated carrot, courgette, or beetroot to your spaghetti bolognese sauce. Add your favourite vegetables to home-made curries.

- Add stir-fried chopped vegetables such as, peppers, courgettes, mushrooms, onions or carrots to ready-made tomato or curry sauces.

- Serve processed foods (such as meat pie) with lots fresh vegetables, such as carrots and cabbage, for a more balanced, nutritious meal.

- Serve pizza with salad or homemade coleslaw.

- Add fresh fruit to rice pudding/ice cream.

- Add a handful of berries, or chopped fruit to yoghurt, or hot/cold custard, for a quick, healthy pudding.

- Add halved strawberries, or slices of melon, mango, or orange, to salads.

Beneficial bug boosters

Some foods contain carbohydrates known as inulins, which feed and stimulate the growth of existing good bacteria in the gut. These are known as prebiotics. They occur naturally in artichokes, onions, garlic, leeks, tomatoes, celery, cucumber, bananas, chickpeas, sunflower seeds, and honey. The benefits of eating these foods include better digestive health, increased immunity, and improved absorption of calcium.

Get fresh

Ideally fruit and vegetables are best eaten as fresh as possible. Storing them properly helps to retain nutrients for longer. It's best not to wash them before putting them in the fridge, as they have a natural coating that helps retain moisture and freshness; washing and scrubbing damages the coating and makes them perish sooner. They also last longer when stored whole. Most vegetables are best stored in perforated plastic or paper bags to help retain moisture – though potatoes are best stored in a cool, dark, dry place.

Carbs – complex and simple!

Carbohydrates are a good source of energy, because they can be converted into glucose more easily than proteins or fats. There are two types of carbohydrate – complex and simple. Complex carbohydrates include cereals, breads, pastas, potatoes, and legumes. They provide a slower, steadier release of energy than simple carbohydrates. Refined carbohydrates, such as white bread and white rice, convert into glucose quicker than whole grains. Carbohydrates should make up about one third of your food intake.

The low-down on sugar

Sugars are simple carbohydrates. There are two main types of sugars, monosaccharides and di-saccharides. Monosaccharides consist of a single sugar molecule and include glucose, fructose, galactose, and fucose. Glucose is found in fruit and vegetables, whilst fructose is found in fruits and honey, and galactose is part of lactose, found in milk and milk products. Fucose is found in vegetables such as mushrooms, and in kelp.

Disaccharides are sugars composed of two linked up monosaccharide molecules and include sucrose, lactose, and maltose. Sucrose is the refined sugar commonly used in foods and drinks. It's extracted from sugar cane and sugar beet and contains both glucose and fructose. Lactose is found in milk and is made up of glucose and galactose. Maltose is formed when sugars are broken down – for example during beer and whisky production, and is made up of two glucose molecules.

Sugar cravings explained

We crave sweet and starchy foods because the glucose they supply provides vital fuel for both brain and body. When our blood sugar is low, a bar of chocolate or a bag of sweets provides a quick burst of energy. This is because sucrose converts quickly into glucose, which is rapidly absorbed into the bloodstream. When the blood sugar rises too high too quickly, the body reacts by producing insulin, which lowers it by directing glucose to the body's cells. Our blood sugar then plummets and we crave another sugar 'hit'. Studies suggest that sugar is addictive and needs to be reduced gradually to prevent withdrawal-type symptoms, such as anxiety.

Sweet enough!

For health and weight management, it's recommended that no more than 10% of our energy should come from sugar. There are 20 calories in 5g (1tsp) sugar, so for a woman this amounts to 50g (10tsp) per day. For a man this equates to 62.5g (12.5tsp).

Curb the cravings

To beat sugar cravings try sniffing a bottle of vanilla essence. Many find it reduces the urge to eat sweet foods. But eating a diet rich in whole grains, rather than refined foods, is the best way to curb sugar cravings.

Sugar – not so sweet!

Over-consumption of sugary foods has been linked to obesity, type 2 diabetes, heart disease, and stroke, as well as tooth decay, gum disease, and ageing skin.

As we've already seen, too much sugar in the diet leads to high blood sugar. This in turn leads to a higher risk of type 2 diabetes.

People who eat a lot of sugar tend to have a low intake of important nutrients, such as vitamins A and C, folic acid, vitamin B12, calcium, phosphorous, magnesium, and iron. Filling up on sugary foods seems to leave less appetite, or room, for more nutritious foods.

A high consumption of sugar and refined carbohydrates can also result in chromium deficiency. Chromium helps to regulate blood sugar and metabolise fats and carbohydrates. It's found in eggs, meats, seafood, whole grains, fruit, and vegetables.

Natural sweeteners

By contrast, natural sugars found in fruit and vegetables are more complex and are absorbed into the bloodstream more slowly. They're essential for various physiological processes, including immune response and brain function.

For a balanced diet, keep sugary foods and drinks to a minimum. This means avoiding eating too many foods containing refined sugar, such as sugar-coated breakfast cereals, sweet biscuits, cakes, and puddings. Research reveals that manufacturers are adding twice as much sugar to some products than 30 years ago. It's also important to avoid sugary drinks such as cola and lemonade, which can contain up to 35g (7tsp) of sugar per 330ml (½pt) bottle! Sugar is even added to savoury foods, such as soups and sauces.

A diet rich in fruit and vegetables will supply sugars in their natural form, along with other nutrients, whereas sucrose has no nutritional value.

Quick tip

SWEETNESS AND LIGHT

If you have a sweet tooth, try to satisfy it with dried fruits, such as raisins, sultanas, dates, figs, prunes, and dried apricots. Fresh fruits, such as ripe bananas, melons, and strawberries are also surprisingly sweet. Once you become accustomed to their natural sweetness, you'll probably find sugary confectionery, cakes, biscuits, and desserts too sweet and cloying.

A.k.a. sugar

When checking food labels for the sugar content of foods, you need to be aware of the other guises it comes under. Any of the following terms indicate added sugars. The main ingredients always come first, so if you notice any of these near the top of the list, you know the sugar content is likely to be high.

- Sucrose
- Glucose
- Glucose syrup
- Fructose
- High fructose corn syrup
- Maltose
- Malt extract
- Hydrolyzed starch
- Invert sugar
- Corn syrup
- Honey
- Dextrose
- Syrup
- Golden syrup
- Treacle

Sugar savers

- Reduce sugar in tea and other beverages gradually, until you can do without.
- Use cinnamon or nutmeg to flavour desserts instead.
- Replace sugar-coated breakfast cereals with whole grain cereals or porridge.
- Freeze a banana on a stick for a sweet, but healthy, alternative to ice cream.
- Choose tinned fruits in natural juice rather than syrup.
- Instead of sweet or stodgy puddings, choose baked apples, summer pudding, or natural yogurt with dried fruit.
- Use reduced-sugar jams.
- When baking, cut the amount of sugar you use by up to half.

Fill up on fibre

High-fibre foods such as whole wheat bread, pasta, rice, and fruit and vegetables, fill you up quicker and for longer, tend to be lower in calories, and speed up weight loss, because your body burns fat to metabolise fibre.

There are two types of fibre – soluble and insoluble. Both types help to lower blood sugar. Soluble fibre does so by slowing down glucose absorption. Soluble fibre can be partially digested and is found mainly in oats, beas, peas, lentils, apples, pears, and strawberries. It's thought to lower cholesterol by absorbing it like a sponge, helping to prevent coronary heart disease. Soluble fibre also acts as a prebiotic, which means it stimulates the growth and activity of beneficial bacteria in the gut. Experts believe this might help relieve inflammatory bowel diseases such as Crohn's disease, ulcerative colitis, and clostidrium difficile, a bacterial infection that causes diarrhoea and colitis. It also keeps blood sugar levels stable, by slowing down the rate at which glucose is absorbed into the bloodstream.

Insoluble fibre can't be digested. It helps other food and waste products move through the gut more easily, thus helping to prevent constipation. This fibre is mainly found in whole grain cereals, brown rice, beans, peas, lentils, oats, fruit and vegetables. It's recommended we eat 18–30g (½–1oz) of fibre daily to enjoy these health benefits.

Fibre providers

To help you eat 18–30g (½–1oz) of fibre a day, here are examples of foods that provide approximately 5g (1/8oz) of fibre. In all cases whole grain versions of cereals, pastas, and rice provide the most fibre. The skins of fruit and vegetables are particularly high in insoluble fibre, so eat them whenever possible.

Where appropriate I've compared the amount you'd need to eat of the white, refined version, to gain the same amount of fibre.

- 2 Weetabix – you'd need to eat 4 x 30g (1oz) servings of cornflakes for the same amount of fibre!

- 2 slices wholemeal bread – you'd have to eat 6 slices of white bread.

- 3 Ryvitas.

- 150g (5oz) brown rice (uncooked) – you'd need to eat 8 times as much white rice for the same amount of fibre!

- 80g (2½oz) whole wheat pasta (uncooked) – you'd need to eat around 3 times this amount of white pasta for the equivalent amount of fibre!

- 1 medium baked potato (180g or 6oz) – including skin. You'd need to eat over twice as much mashed potato.

- One third of a 415g (14oz) tin of baked beans.

- Half a cup of cooked sweetcorn.

- 2 medium oranges, pears, apples, or bananas.

- 45g (3 tablespoons) of frozen peas.

FIBRE AND FOOD LABELS

Current guidelines suggest that a food labelled 'High Fibre' should contain 6g of fibre per 100g (¼oz per 4oz). A food labelled 'a source of fibre' should contain 3g of fibre per 100g (1/8oz per 4oz).

Fibre benefits

A diet high in fibre, offers numerous health benefits. These include reducing the risk of constipation, piles, diverticular disease, cancers of the bowel and colon, breast cancer in pre-menopausal women, type 2 diabetes, and coronary heart disease.

Building blocks of life

Protein is necessary for the growth of cells and repair of tissues. All proteins comprise different combinations of 20 compounds known as amino acids. Depending on the amino acids they contain, proteins form enzymes, hormones, muscles, organs, and other tissues in the body.

There are two types of amino acids:

- non-essential amino acids – which the body can make.
- essential amino acids – which the body can't make and therefore must be obtained from food.

Protein types

Animal proteins – which contain all the essential amino acids and are found in meat, poultry, fish, eggs, dairy products.

Plant proteins – which contain various amino acids. Sources of plant protein include pulses, cereals, grains, nuts and seeds, soya and Quorn – made with vegetable protein obtained from fungus. No one source contains all the essential amino acids, so if you're vegetarian you need to eat a mix of these foods. For example, beans on toast, or cereal with milk.

Quick tip

RED MEAT ALERT
Research has linked a high intake of red and processed meats, such as sausages and burgers, to a greater risk of stomach, bowel, and breast cancers. Plant proteins are low in fat and high in fibre, vitamins, minerals, and phytochemicals linked to good health and the prevention of illness; so it's best to eat more plant proteins than animal ones.

Protein requirements

It's recommended that we get between 10% and 15% of our daily energy intake from protein. This translates into roughly 50g–75g (2oz–2½oz) for women and 65g–95g (2¼oz–3½oz) for men.

Protein providers

To give you an idea of what you'd need to eat to get your recommended daily amounts here's the approximate protein content of some everyday foods:

- One medium egg – 6g (¼oz) of protein.
- One skinless chicken breast (130g/4½oz) – 40g (1¼oz) of protein.
- One small fillet steak (200g/7oz) – 50g (1¾oz) of protein.
- One beef burger, or pork sausage – 8g (1/3oz) of protein.
- One portion of poached skinless cod fillet (150g/5oz) – 30g (1oz) of protein.
- Half a can of tuna – 20g (½oz) of protein.
- One portion of cheese (50g/1¾oz) – 12g (½oz) of protein.
- One tablespoon of boiled red lentils (40g/1oz) – 3g (1/8oz) of protein.
- One portion of tofu (125g/4½oz) – 15g (½oz) of protein.
- One medium slice wholemeal bread – 4g (1/6oz) of protein.
- One medium slice white bread – 3g (1/8oz) of protein.
- 150ml (1/3pt) glass of milk – 5g (1/8oz) of protein.

Do dairy

Eat low-fat dairy foods, such as cheese and yogurt, for health benefits linked to their protein and calcium content. Recent research revealed that those who include dairy foods in a weight loss regime lose more weight than those who don't – particularly around the waistline. There are several likely reasons for this. One is that the protein in dairy foods produces a feeling of fullness and stabilises the blood sugar, reducing sugar cravings and the urge to snack. Another is that milk sugar—lactose—keeps the blood sugar steady, because it converts into glucose more slowly than sucrose.

Also the high calcium content reduces the amount of fat absorbed from foods. Calcium even appears to speed up the rate at which calories are burned.

These benefits appear to halve the risk of developing insulin resistance, a condition where the body doesn't respond properly to insulin. Insulin resistance can result from prolonged high blood sugar levels. It leads to increased cholesterol levels, blood pressure and fat storage, and raises the risk of heart disease, type 2 diabetes, and stroke.

Calcium, along with vitamin D, is also necessary for strong bones and the prevention of osteoporosis. Plus it promotes serenity and aids sleep. Studies show it helps prevent PMT and might also ease menopausal symptoms.

The current recommendation is that men and women obtain at least 700mg (1/5oz) of calcium daily from their diet. This equates to roughly 500ml (1 pint) of milk, 3 small tubs of plain or fruit yogurt, or around 100g (4oz) of hard cheese.

Fat facts

When it comes to eating more healthily and losing weight, most people consider cutting down on the fat content of their diet. Whilst fats are high in energy—1g (1/16oz) provides 9 kcal, compared to 4 kcal in 1g (1/16oz) of carbohydrate or protein—they are necessary for good health. They're needed for various important functions, including the transportation and absorption of fat-soluble vitamins A, D, E, and K, and the cushioning of vital organs. Fats lubricate our skin and gut and help to make food more appetising too. They also make food more filling because they slow down glucose absorption – so adding small amounts of beneficial fats can actually help weight management. However, whilst some fats are essential to good health, others are detrimental. Too much of any fat can lead to weight gain. So it's important to ensure you get the correct amounts of the right types of fat.

Healthy fats

The healthiest fats are unsaturated. There are two types of unsaturated fat – polyunsaturated essential fatty acids (Omegas 3 and 6) and monounsaturated fat (Omega 9).

Essential fatty acids—EFAs—are fats that can't be made by the body and are needed for various functions, including eyesight, healthy skin, hair and nails, and brain function.

Omega 3s are anti-inflammatory and anti-coagulant and essential for brain development and function. They help protect against cardiovascular disease, arthritis, skin complaints, Huntington's Disease, and Multiple Sclerosis. They also appear to help prevent and treat ADHD, dyslexia, depression, and other mood disorders and schizophrenia. Health experts recently recommended that all pupils should be given fish oils to reduce disruptive behaviour and improve learning.

Good sources of Omega 3s are:

- Oily fish – pilchards, sardines, salmon, mackerel.
- Nuts – especially walnuts, Brazil nuts, and almonds.
- Seeds – especially sesame.
- Oils including soya bean, sunflower, canola, rapeseed.
- Egg yolks.

Omega 6s are also anti-inflammatory and can help prevent and treat a range of conditions; they can ease the symptoms of IBS and promote healthy skin, hair, and nails. They promote hormonal balance – relieving and preventing PMT and menopausal symptoms.

Omega 6 fatty acids are found in:

- Sunflower and corn oils.
- Some vegetables and grains.
- Nuts & seeds.
- Olives.

Most people in the UK get enough of these in their diet.

Monounsaturated, or **Omega-9**, fats can lower bad, LDL, cholesterol and increase good, HDL, cholesterol.

Good sources of Omega-9 fats are:

- Olives and olive oil.
- Peanut oil.
- Nuts – especially almonds and Brazil nuts.
- Seeds – particularly sesame seeds.
- Rapeseed oil.
- Avocados.

…. and fats to avoid

Saturated fats, otherwise known as hard fats, and mainly found in animal products such as red meat, butter and full-fat dairy foods, such as cheese and milk. Too much saturated fat can raise bad LDL cholesterol levels, which increases the risk of heart disease and atherosclerosis. It might also be linked to some cancers, including breast cancer.

Trans fats, also known as partially hydrogenated oils, which are mainly found in processed foods. These are formed when liquid vegetable oils are turned into solid fats, through a process called hydrogenation. Trans fats might be even more detrimental to health than saturated fats. One 6-year study showed that monkeys who were fed a diet where 8% of the calories came from trans fats, gained about a fourteenth of their body weight, compared with monkeys fed the same diet – but with monounsaturated fats, such as olive oil, replacing the trans fats, who gained less than a fiftieth. The monkeys eating trans fats also carried about a third more fat on their stomachs, which is a risk factor for heart disease and diabetes.

Reduce saturated and trans fats and increase polyunsaturated and monounsaturated fats in your diet by:

- Choosing lean meat and trimming off visible fat. Removing the skin from roast chicken.
- Grilling, baking, poaching, stea microwaving, rather than frying or roasting.
- Skimming off any fat that rises to the top ooking stews, or mince.
- Adding more vegetables and less meat to stews/c s.

- Choosing a low-fat accompaniment to a high-fat food, such as meat pie or pizza, e.g. steamed vegetables, or salad, to achieve a more balanced meal.
- Selecting ready meals with a lower fat content – check the label; 3% of food = low fat, 20% = high fat.
- Measuring oil when cooking, rather than guessing.
- Using a low-fat spread preferably made with olive oil, rather than butter or full-fat margarine.
- Opting for lower-fat dairy foods, such as low-fat yogurts, reduced fat cheeses and semi-skimmed or skimmed milk.
- Grating cheese, so you use less.
- Avoiding products with hydrogenated fat, hydrogenated vegetable oil, partially hydrogenated vegetable fat/oil or trans fatty acids listed in the ingredients.
- Avoiding products with animal/saturated fats, shortening, glycerides, palm oils, and milk fats listed in the ingredients.
- Choosing margarines labelled 'low in trans' or 'virtually trans free'.
- Eating oily fish 3 times a week.
- Snacking on a handful of nuts or seeds.
- Eat hummus – it contains sesame seed paste.
- Using olive oil as a salad dressing and in cooking.
- Mashing potato with olive oil, rather than milk and butter.
- Using herbs like basil, mint, or coriander and strong condiments such as mustard, soy sauce and balsamic or white wine vinegar to flavour foods, rather than high-fat sauces and mayonnaises.

Quick tip

FATS ENOUGH!

Remember, all fats are high in calories, so to ensure a balanced diet and to help maintain a healthy weight it's recommended that no more than a third of our daily energy intake should come from fats. This translates into about 75g (2½oz) for women, of which no more than 20g (¾oz) should be saturated fat, and 90g (3¼oz) for men, of which no more than 30g (1oz) should be saturated fats.

Swap shop

An easy way to reduce the fat content in your diet is to swap your favourite treats for lower fat, less calorific versions. Here are some ideas to get you started:

- Swap fried or scrambled eggs, for poached or boiled eggs.
- Swap pan-fried chips for oven chips.
- Swap Greek yoghurt for low-fat plain yoghurt. Low-fat natural set yoghurt has a deceptively creamy texture.
- Swap chocolate cake for low-fat chocolate mousse.
- Swap a bag of crisps for sugar-free popcorn.
- Swap ice cream for fruit sorbet.
- Swap a croissant for a toasted bagel, with low fat spread.
- Swap cheddar cheese for Edam.

Seasonal swaps

Christmas is a time of indulgence, but it's still possible to party and eat more healthily!

- Swap a sausage roll for a cocktail sausage.
- Swap a handful of salted peanuts for 10 olives.
- Swap a slice of cheesecake for a portion of pavlova.
- Swap a cheese straw for a breadstick.
- Swap guacamole for salsa.
- Swap Brie for Stilton.

Plan for health

Plan your menu for the week ahead before you shop. This helps you achieve a healthier diet, because you can decide beforehand which foods you need to buy, rather than grabbing anything that catches your eye. It's much easier to eat a balanced diet if the right ingredients are in the cupboard.

Ready, steady, cook!

Processed foods and ready meals tend to contain more unhealthy fats, sugar and salt. Try preparing meals from basic ingredients for healthier meals. Not only are they more nutritious, they're also far tastier. Try adapting recipes to make them healthier: grill, bake, steam, boil, or microwave instead of frying. Use wholemeal flour, or part wholemeal flour, instead of white. Substitute herbs for salt. Experiment with reducing the amount of sugar in desserts and baking. Some recipes work well with up to half the suggested amount.

No time to cook?

Preparing a healthy meal needn't take a long time. Try roasting vegetables such as peppers, tomatoes, onions, and courgettes with garlic and herbs. Add to cooked whole wheat pasta and stir in a low-fat cream alternative. You could add tuna, or Parmesan for added protein. Stir-fries only take minutes to prepare and cook. Broths and casseroles are easy to make – you can do other jobs, once they're on the hob or in the oven. For extra speed, substitute frozen vegetables for fresh. Make your own healthier versions of ready meals by cooking extra portions of your favourite dishes and freezing them.

Eating out

For more balanced eating out, always opt for small portion sizes. Don't be tempted by the super-size portions on offer in many fast-food outlets. Fill up with salad – most restaurants offer salads as starters or side dishes. Don't be frightened to ask for alternatives to foods on the menu. For example, ask if you can have a baked potato, rather than chips, or vegetables and fish, such as tuna or prawns, as a pizza topping.

If you crave something sweet, order a dessert to share, rather than one all to yourself. You'll still satisfy your sweet tooth – only with half the fat and sugar. You'll probably find that after eating possibly a starter and main course, half a dessert is enough. Or swap a starter for dessert, or vice versa.

Focus on eating slowly – especially if your restaurant's décor is brightly coloured! Studies suggest lurid colour schemes encourage people to eat faster and consequently eat more.

Dining out dos & don'ts

Choose dishes containing the least fat when eating out.

At an Indian restaurant

Many dishes contain a lot of oil or ghee—which is clarified butter—so you need to choose wisely. Avoid deep-fried starters like onion bhajis and samosas. Poppadoms are lower in fat. Lime pickle is high in fat and mango chutney is high in sugar. Opt instead for raita (cucumber dip) or tomato sambai (tomato and onion dip) as an accompaniment.

Forgo creamy curries such as korma, masala or passanda and opt for tandoori, tikka, or madras dishes, with boiled rice and chapatti, rather than pilau rice and naan, which are quite high in fat. Other lower-fat dishes include aloo gobi, vegetable curry and aloo saag.

At an Italian restaurant

Eat dishes with tomato- rather than cream-based sauces, and choose lower-fat pizza toppings such as vegetables, prawns, or ham. Instead of garlic bread, try bruschetta – a ciabatta bread with a tomato and herb topping.

In a Chinese Restaurant

Avoid foods in batter, as they're high in fat. Go for lower-fat options, such as stir-fries with boiled rice or noodles, chicken chop suey or Szechuan dishes.

In a Thai restaurant

Again avoid battered foods. Choose stir-fried or steamed dishes with jasmine rice, rather than egg-fried. Thai green and red curries contain coconut milk, which is low in calories but high in saturated fat, and could therefore contribute to high cholesterol or heart disease, so eat them in moderation.

At a Japanese restaurant

Choose sushi and stir-fries. Again avoid battered dishes such as tempura. Japanese banquets tend to consist of small portions of various foods including salads, fish, chicken, and miso soups, and on the whole provide a fairly healthy and balanced cuisine.

At a Mexican restaurant

Select salsa with fajitas, rather than sour cream. Salsa is low in fat and contains phytonutrients.

Better burgers and kebabs

At a burger bar choose grilled rather than fried and opt for those made from lean meat or fish. Say "no" to cheese or mayonnaise and ask for a wholemeal bun and extra salad. If you enjoy a kebab go for chicken rather than lamb, which is much fattier. Add salad and chilli sauce, rather than garlic mayonnaise, for a lower-fat and more balanced meal.

At a fish & chip shop

To make fish and chips a healthier option, don't eat all of the batter, as it soaks up a lot of fat, or go for fish in breadcrumbs, which absorbs less fat. Try a smaller portion of chips, or share them. Another tip is to blot the fat from your meal using kitchen roll. But be aware that fried fish and chips are high in fat and are best eaten only occasionally if you're serious about being healthy. Or you could forgo the fish shop altogether and opt for the lower-fat alternative of oven baked frozen chips and oven baked fish in breadcrumbs. Serve with peas, green beans, or broad beans for a more nutritious meal. Finally, avoid adding salt if you can. But go ahead with the traditional sprinkling of vinegar, because it helps you absorb certain minerals and keeps your blood sugar steady.

Healthier sandwiches

Choose brown, granary, or wholemeal bread for extra fibre. Select low-fat fillings such as lean meat, tuna, prawns, hard boiled egg, or cheese such as Edam, Emmental, Gruyere, or low fat cream cheese. For extra vitamins go for added salad. If the sandwich is made to order, opt for no, or only a little, butter, margarine, or mayonnaise, or for lower-fat versions. Avoid full-fat mayonnaise, choose low-fat salad dressings, salsa, or mustard instead.

When buying pre-packed sandwiches, check the label for the fat content. Choose sandwiches with 3% of fat and 1% saturated fat, or less if possible.

Saline solution

A high intake of salt is linked with high blood pressure and the risk of coronary heart disease, stroke, stomach cancer, osteoporosis, kidney problems, and even stomach ulcers. Government guidelines urge us to eat no more than 6g (¼oz) of salt daily, but this can be hard to achieve if you eat a lot of processed and pre-packaged foods. For example, pre-packed sandwiches can contain between 2.5g (1/16oz) and 4g (1/6oz) of salt and a tin of a well-known brand's 'healthy' lentil and bacon soup contains 4g (1/6oz). A 400g (14oz) tin of regular baked beans contains 5g (1/8oz) of salt.

Doctors claim that 35,000 lives could be saved each year if we all stuck to the recommended limit. The best way to reduce salt in your diet is to eat meals prepared and cooked at home, using little or no salt.

Try flavouring your cooking with herbs. Use lime, garlic, ginger, and chillis in stir-fries. Squeeze lemon juice on fish and seafood. Use black pepper on pasta and eggs. Olives and pickled capers are also good for adding flavour to pastas, pizzas, and salads.

When cooking from scratch isn't possible, check food labels for salt content. But beware, many food manufacturers give the sodium content, which has to be multiplied by 2.5 to calculate the salt content. Plus, the sodium or salt content per 100g (3½oz) is often provided, which again necessitates arithmetic to work out the total amount in a product.

Products listing any of the following among their ingredients are likely to be high in salt:

- Monosodium glutamate.
- Disodium phosphate.
- Brine.
- Garlic salt.
- Onion salt.
- Sodium benzoate.
- Sodium alginate.
- Sodium hydroxide.
- Sodium caseinate.
- Sodium hydroxide.
- Sodium nitrate.
- Sodium pectinate.
- Sodium propionate.
- Sodium sulphite.
- Soy sauce.
- Baking powder.
- Baking soda.

Hidden extras

Many processed foods are high in added sugar, fat, or salt — all of which can lead to weight gain and health problems.

Food labels – a quick & easy guide

	Amount per 100g	
	HIGH	LOW
Total fat	20g	3g
Saturated fat	5g	1g
Sugar	10g	2g
Salt	1.5g	0.3g
Sodium	0.5g	0.1g

Ingredients, including additives, have to be listed in descending order of weight, so it's easy to spot the main ones.

Read the label

Low-fat products often contain excessive amounts of added sugar. For example, a yogurt containing only 2.7g of fat per 100g is labelled low-fat, suggesting it's a healthy food choice. Yet it contains 15.7g of sugar per 100g – 19.6 g per pot, which equals nearly 4 teaspoons!

Breakfast cereals are viewed as a healthy start to the day, yet they're often high in sugar, salt and fat. A well-known supermarket's own-brand crunchy oat cereal contains 20.3g of fat per 100g – proving it really does pay to read the label!

Some savoury sauces and pizzas contain added sugar.

It's best to choose foods with as few additives as possible. For example natural unsweetened yogurt – you can add dried fruit to sweeten it, if necessary. Plain porridge oats, or shredded wheat, have no hidden extras so are a healthier choice.

But don't be misled!

Food labels can be very misleading. Here's a brief guide to commonly used terms and what they actually mean.

Strawberry flavour doesn't mean a product contains strawberries, however strawberry flavoured does. Also, if there's a picture of strawberries on the wrapper, the item must contain them. But check the label, as the strawberry content could be very low.

Words such as original, healthy, authentic, wholesome, nutritious, selected, and real, mean nothing at all, as there is no legal definition for them.

Light or 'lite' doesn't mean a product is low in fat. It usually means the product is lower in fat than the standard version, but it could still contain more fat than the standard version from another brand.

Reduced fat doesn't mean low fat. The term can be used to describe a food that contains 25% less fat than the standard version. The food could still be high in fat. The same applies to reduced sugar, sodium, and energy! Often a reduced fat product has added sugar to make it more palatable, so the calories it contains remain the same as the standard version.

Fat-free doesn't equal low in fat. For example if a product states it's 92 per cent fat free, that means it contains 8 per cent fat, which makes it a medium-fat food.

Natural, or made from natural, simply means that the manufacturer made the product using ingredients from a natural source. After processing, these ingredients may bear little resemblance to their original state!

Free from artificial preservatives might mean a product contains other additives that extend shelf life, such as salt or sugar.

Farm fresh, or country fresh eggs, might bear an image of a hen scratching around a farmyard, but in all likelihood, they'll have been produced by battery hens. Free-range eggs must come from hens with access to the outdoors. Barn eggs come from hens that live indoors, but have freedom of movement and access to perches and nests. Organic eggs are guaranteed to have been laid by uncaged hens, allowed to roam on organic pasture.

STOP AT THE TRAFFIC LIGHTS!

Many food manufacturers now use traffic light colours on the front of food products to help you identify if the food has low, medium, or high levels of fat, sugar, and salt. Green indicates low, amber medium, and red high. So the more green lights on a product, the healthier it is, in terms of fat, sugar, and salt levels.

Choosing foods with amber lights is OK most of the time, if you balance them with some mainly green light ones. Eat foods with red lights in small amounts, or as occasional treats to keep a healthy balance. If you're choosing between similar items, go for the one with the most greens and ambers for the healthiest option.

Guideline Daily Amounts

Some food companies use this system, which displays the calories and grams of sugars, fats, and salt, in a serving of food and how this measures up as a percentage of your Guideline Daily Amounts.

But the figures given are often for servings much smaller than are usually eaten. Also, the percentages are usually calculated against the dietary needs of an adult man, which are different from those of women, teenagers, and children.

Smart snacking

Do you often hit an energy slump mid-morning or afternoon and reach for the biscuit tin, a chocolate bar, or bag of crisps? Snacking in itself isn't necessarily a bad thing, depending on the kinds of foods you choose. Junk foods might offer a short-term energy boost, but they're likely to add extra fat, sugar, and salt to your diet and few nutrients. If you eat nutritious snacks, they help to maintain your blood sugar levels and provide valuable vitamins, minerals, and fibre. Whether at home or at work, always make sure you have a selection of healthy foods to graze on. Fresh fruit, dried fruit, nuts, seeds, carrot or celery sticks, oat cakes, plain digestives, natural yoghurt, cottage cheese, crispbreads with peanut butter or hummus, nut or muesli bars and malt loaf, are all excellent snack foods.

Let your medicine
be your food
and your food
be your medicine.

Hippocrates

Super foods, herbs & spices

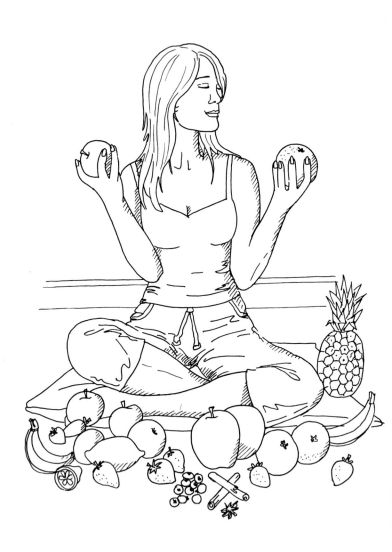

chapter 4
Superfoods, herbs & spices

Superfoods deliver a high concentration of health-boosting nutrients. However, remember the key to a healthy diet is to eat a variety of foods. If your current diet is based on processed foods, you'll reap huge health benefits by gradually introducing some of them. None are expensive or exotic – they are everyday items that can be bought at your local supermarket.

Studies confirm that ancient claims about the health-giving properties of herbs are more than just folklore. Many contain higher concentrations of antioxidants than fruit and vegetables and have anti-bacterial properties. They also contain phytochemicals and vitamins. Whilst we tend to consume herbs in small amounts, they nevertheless offer a tasty way to improve health.

Some herbs make pleasant-tasting infusions. Use 2 teaspoons of fresh herbs, or 1 teaspoon of dried herbs per cup of boiling water. Pour the boiling water over the herb, cover and leave to stand for five to ten minutes. Strain and add honey to taste. Drink whilst hot.

Spices are usually extracted from the bark, stem and seeds of plants. They add flavour to food, and offer health benefits when consumed regularly. Even a pinch is enough to make a difference, because of the potent chemicals they contain – such as isothiocyanates – natural compounds which seem to inhibit cancers.

A handful of almonds

Eating a handful of almonds daily reduces CHD, cancer and diabetes risk factors and has an anti-ageing effect. Almonds contain 20 flavonoids, vitamin E and monounsaturated fat, as well as protein, fibre and minerals. Flavanoids have an antioxidant effect on the body, protecting cells from damage and preventing clogged arteries. Almonds also appear to boost weight loss. The protein, fat and fibre keep you full longer and not all of the calories they contain are absorbed, because of their tough cell walls. Finally, almonds are good for your bones, as they are rich in calcium.

Red hot chilli peppers

High in vitamin A and the anti-oxidant beta carotene, chilli peppers also contain capsaicin, which gives them their heat, and may stop the spread of prostrate and pancreatic cancer cells. Capsaicin also prevents and treats stomach ulcers, because it reduces acid and increases alkali, as well as improving blood circulation in the stomach. Excessive amounts of hot chillies has been linked to stomach cancer, so don't overdo them.

Chilli peppers seem to keep blood insulin levels steady, so may reduce the risk of type 2 diabetes.

Consuming dishes containing chilli regularly helps burn fat cells and raise the metabolism. Chillis are also anti-inflammatory, bringing relief to arthritis sufferers, and may help prevent atherosclerosis. Chillis stimulate the release of 'feel good' brain chemicals, endorphins, which also have a pain-relieving effect.

An apple a day …

An apple a day does indeed keep the doctor away. They appear to act as 'magic bullets' against various cancers, as well as reduce blood cholesterol and provide vitamins and minerals. Apples contain quercetin, which belongs to a group of plant pigments known as a flavonoids. Quercetin is an antioxidant which boosts the immune system, helping to reduce the risk of illnesses ranging from the common cold, to breast, colon and prostate cancers and heart disease. The skins contain phytonutrients known to reduce the growth of colon cancer cells by 43%.

Eating five or more apples a week can improve lung function and reduce the risk of asthma in adults. Children whose mothers eat apples during pregnancy are less likely to develop asthma. This may be down to the antioxidants counteracting the effects of pollution and easing inflammation.

Apples also contain pectin, a soluble fibre which mops up cholesterol. Crunching into an apple cleans between your teeth and massages your gums, promoting dental health. Finally, fresh apples are a decent source of vitamin C and, because of their low glycaemic index, help you to maintain a healthy weight.

Go bananas

Bananas provide energy and protect against strokes, heart disease, stomach ulcers and anaemia, as well as reducing stress and depression. They're high in potassium, which helps maintain sodium levels in the body and prevent high blood pressure. They also contain tryptophan and vitamin B6, which are used by the body to make mood-enhancing serotonin.

Berry good for you !

Berries such as blueberries, blackberries, blackcurrants, cranberries, raspberries and strawberries, are a rich source of health-promoting vitamins, minerals and phytochemicals.

They're rich in vitamins C and E and anthocyanins, powerful antioxidants, which are anti-ageing, anti-cardiovascular disease, anti-cancer and antibacterial. Anthocyanins are plant pigments – the darker the fruit, the more it contains, so fruits such as blackcurrants, blueberries and blackberries are rich sources. Cranberries also contain beneficial amounts. A serving of ten strawberries provides the recommended daily allowance of folic acid.

The vitamins and anthocyanins in berries appear to prevent age-related brain deterioration and may improve short-term memory and restore coordination. They may keep eyes healthy, reducing eyestrain, improving night vision and helping to prevent macular degeneration.

Anthocyanins are also effective against E.coli – a common cause of stomach upsets, diarrohea and cystitis. Berries such as blueberries and cranberries also contain a substance which discourages this bacteria from sticking to the mucous membranes of the bladder and uretha, again helping to prevent urinary tract infections. H.pylori, a cause of stomach ulcers, is also prevented from adhering to the stomach lining. Anthocyanins may also prevent the excessive growth of fungi in the body, such as Candida albicans, which often causes vaginal infections and has been linked with IBS. They seems to slow the growth of the bacteria which cause gum disease, helping promote better oral health.

Another antioxidant found in berries, ellagic acid, is believed to prevent cancers, by restricting cancer cell growth. Raspberries contain the highest amounts.

Berries are also rich in the soluble fibre pectin too. Their seeds are beneficial too – providing essential fatty acids. Studies suggest that blackcurrants are the most nutritious berries, followed by blueberries, raspberries and strawberries.

Brain-boosting Brazils

Like other nuts, Brazil nuts are packed with essential vitamins and minerals. They are an excellent source of selenium, believed to protect against Alzheimer's, depression and cancer. Research suggests that eating a few brazil nuts daily can reduce the risk of cancers of the liver, lungs, stomach and prostate.

They're rich in Omega-3 and Omega-6 fatty acids and oleic acid and contain vitamin E which is antioxidant and anti-ageing. They also contain linoleic acid, important for skin/hormone balance.

Quick tip

CARROTS ARE TOPS !
Carrots are a good source of the antioxidant betacarotene. To gain the most benefit, roast carrots in a healthy fat, such as olive oil. Roasting softens the cell walls, making the betacarotene more digestible. Adding fat helps the body to absorb it. Tests also suggest that falcarinol, a natural pesticide in carrots, may lower the risk of cancer. They're also rich in soluble fibre.

Beet it!

Beetroot purifies the blood, boosts immunity and has anti-cancer properties. It's a good source of folic acid, which may protect against Alzheimer's, dementia and high blood pressure and helps maintain a good supply of red blood cells. Folic acid is essential during early pregnancy to prevent spinal cord defects, such as spina bifida. Liver is the best source, but isn't recommended during pregnancy, due to its high levels of vitamin A, which can harm the baby. A 100g serving of beetroot contains 75% of the recommended daily intake. Beetroot also contains iron—again needed for healthy blood and silica—essential for healthy tendons, ligaments, bones, fingernails, skin and hair. Rich in soluble fibre, it has a 'medium' Glycaemic Index.

It's may also lower homocysteine levels in the blood. Homocysteine is an amino acid produced by the body when it breaks down methionine, another amino acid. A high level in the blood indicates a high risk of developing diseases such cardiovascular disease, dementia, osteoporosis and problems in pregnancy. Eating foods rich in folic acid and vitamins B6 & 12 lowers homocysteine to a safer level. Other foods rich in folic acid include green leafy vegetables, citrus fruits, pulses and wholegrain cereals.

Opt for oranges

Oranges are high in vitamin C and the phytonutrient hesperitin, which appears to discourage breast cancer cell growth. Eating oranges and other citrus fruits seems to reduce the risk of both stomach and skin cancers.

DARK CHOCOLATE INDULGENCE

Studies show that good-quality dark chocolate contains flavanols, which are antioxidants with a clot-busting and blood-pressure lowering effect. They also appear to boost blood flow to the brain, improving brain function and counteracting fatigue. Chocolate also increases mood and sleep-enhancing serotonin in the brain. Milk chocolate contains fewer flavanols and more fat and sugar. For maximum health benefits eat about one to two ounces daily, as even dark chocolate can be high in fat and sugar!

Grapes are great!

Eating red or purple grapes could prevent a host of illnesses and even help you sleep better! They contain resveratrol, an antioxidant believed to balance hormones, prevent breast and prostate cancers and osteoporosis, and protect against thrombosis and hardening of the arteries. Other antioxidants in grapes are believed to reduce cholesterol levels, prevent Alzheimer's, gum disease, colds and allergies, and benefit arthritis. Grapes are thought to contain melatonin, a hormone that helps regulate the sleep cycle.

Have hazelnuts

Just fifteen hazelnuts provide the recommended daily intake of vitamin E for women. Vitamin E protects the body from the effects of pollution, stress and the sun. It may also help prevent cataracts and Alzheimer's.

Eat your greens

Green vegetables such as broccoli, Brussels sprouts, cauliflower and cabbage generally contain antioxidant vitamins A and C and vitamin B complex, including folic acid. Folic acid is especially important in early pregnancy.

Dark green vegetables are also rich in vitamin K, which keeps bones strong by regulating calcium levels and promoting blood clotting. Eat dark green vegetables in moderation if you take warfarin to prevent blood clotting, as too much Vitamin K could effect the drug's effectiveness. Broccoli and purple sprouting broccoli are rich in vitamin C. One portion contains the recommended daily amount. It also contains the natural phytoestrogen (plant oestrogen) lignan, believed to protect against breast cancer and relieve menopausal symptoms.

Leafy green vegetables are a good source of iron. Iron comes in two different forms, haem, from meat, and non-haem, from plants. Non-haem is harder for the body to absorb. Vitamin C aids absorption, making leafy green vegetables good for vegetarians and vegans. Broccoli, kale and spinach are also rich in the antioxidants beta-carotene and lutein. Beta-carotene protects against various cancers and UV light. Lutein reduces the risk of age-related macular degeneration, which can lead to blindness. It also protects the eyes from UV damage and cataracts. Eating these vegetables with a small amount of fat, such as olive oil, helps your body absorb the lutein.

Green vegetables are thought to have anti-cancer properties, due to their glucosinolate content. Glucosinolates are compounds containing glucose and sulphur. They give vegetables such as Brussels sprouts their bitter taste.

How we store and cook our greens can have a marked effect on the glucosinolate content.

FRESH BEATS FROZEN
Freezing and thawing green vegetables cuts the glucosinolate content by a third. Storing fresh vegetables in the fridge or at room temperature for a week has little effect.

Slice, don't shred

Finely shredding green vegetables also destroys glucosinolates. So slice or tear instead.

Steam or stir-fry

Boiling green vegetables dramatically lowers the glucosinolate, vitamin C and folic acid content. Microwaving in a little water is better, but steaming and stir-frying preserve the most nutrients.

Know your onions

Like apples, onions contain quercetin, but absorption from onions is three times greater. Like garlic, onions contain good levels of allicin. They're also a good source of chromium, which helps stabilise blood sugar, maintain hormonal balance and prevent PMT. Finally, they're natural pre-biotics, which promote the growth of 'good' bacteria in the gut.

A taste of honey

If you have a sweet tooth, try replacing sugar with honey, which is a healthier alternative, because it contains amino acids, vitamins, minerals and antioxidants. Honey contains a mixture of fructose, glucose, maltose, sucrose and other sugars, formed from nectar by an enzyme produced by bees. A source of natural sugars, it's an instant energy -booster, but has a gentler and longer-lasting effect on blood sugar levels than sugar.

It also provides trace amounts of B vitamins, and minerals, including calcium, iron, zinc, potassium and chromium. The presence selenium, vitamin C , enzymes and flavanoids, gives honey its antioxidant properties. Researchers recently concluded that honey has a mild cholesterol-lowering effect.

If you suffer from hayfever, try eating one teaspoon of honey produced within a five mile radius of where you live, every day. The pollen in the honey will boost your immunity to the allergens that cause your hayfever.

Mushroom magic

Mushrooms seem to lower oestrogen levels, which may help reduce the risk of breast cancer. They may cut the risk of prostate cancer by inhibiting enzymes linked with its development. They're rich in antioxidants and the immunity-boosting trace-mineral selenium. They contain insoluble fibre and a natural statin called lovastatin, both of which lower cholesterol, helping to reduce the risk of CHD. They're also rich in blood-pressure-lowering potassium. Finally, mushrooms are a good source of B vitamins, including folic acid.

Have you had your oats?

Oats contain soluble fibre, called beta glucan, which lowers blood cholesterol, cutting the risk of heart disease. Rich in insoluble fibre, they have a low glycaemic index, making porridge a good breakfast to help manage your weight.
Plus they're a good source of chromium, which balances blood sugar, iron, zinc, manganese, vitamin E, thiamin and folate.

Not just cool for cats!

Oily fish such as salmon, sardines, herrings, mackerel, trout and tuna are high in protein and contain up to eight times as much health-boosting omega-3 and omega-6 fatty acids as lean fish, such as cod, haddock, monkfish and sole.

Sprats contain the most, followed by salmon, pilchards, mackerel and herring. Fresh tuna and trout are also decent sources, rich in vitamin E and selenium. Canned oily fish with edible bones, such as salmon and sardines, are a good source of calcium too.

Love olive oil

Olive oil features heavily in the Mediterranean diet which is believed to reduce the risk of heart disease, stroke and cancer. It's rich in monounsaturated fats, which lower blood cholesterol and a good source of Vitamin E, which thins the blood, boosts immunity and acts as an antioxidant. Evidence that it reduces the risk of breast, skin and colon cancer is attributed to other components, such as oleic acid and phenols. It has a sweet, slightly spicy flavour and is great as a dip for fresh crusty brown bread, or as a salad dressing.

Peanut power

Peanuts contain soluble and non-soluble fibre, good for the digestion and lowering cholesterol. They're high in protein and a good source of polyunsaturated and monounsaturated fats. More than 75 percent of the total fat content is unsaturated. They contain the amino acid arginine, resveratrol (also found in red wine), plant sterols and other phytochemicals which are thought to have cardio-protective and cancer-preventing properties. They're cholesterol free and contain minerals such as zinc, magnesium, copper and selenium, plus vitamin Bs, folate and vitamin E. Eating peanut butter seems to aid weight loss – probably because of its low glycaemic index. For the healthiest option, choose a variety without hydrogenated fat.

THE HUMBLE POTATO

Potatoes are cheap, filling, nutritious and low in fat, if you bake or boil them and don't add too much butter or margarine. They contain carbohydrate, protein and fibre. They're also a good source of B vitamins, including B6 and folic acid and provide vitamin C.

Sweet potato sustenance

Sweet potatoes are even more nutritious than white potatoes and have a lower Glycaemic Index, so they keep you full for longer. They contain the antioxidant betacarotene and three times as much vitamin C as a regular potato.

Take your pulse

Pulses include beans, peas and lentils. They have anti-cancer properties; a compound they contain inhibits an enzyme linked to tumour growth. A good source of protein, slow-release carbohydrate, soluble and insoluble fibre, vitamins and minerals, pulses are a valuable addition to anyone's diet. They also count as one portion of vegetables.

Haricot beans, otherwise known as baked beans are an excellent source of iron, folic acid and calcium. For the healthiest option, go for the low salt and sugar versions.

Red kidney beans, an ingredient of the popular mexican dish, chilli con carne, contain a substance which can upset the stomach. Either boil for fifteen minutes and then drain before use, or for ease, use the tinned versions.

Soya beans supply all of the essential amino acids, making them the only source of first class plant protein. They're also the best food source of isoflavones, plant hormones which reduce menopausal symptoms and the risk of breast cancer in women. Soya also reduces the risk of prostate and colon cancers and lowers cholesterol.

Peas also contain fibre and lutein, an antioxidant believed to protect eye health.

Lentils are high in fibre—a 200g portion contains around 16g —almost the recommended daily amount.

Peas also contain fibre, slow-release carbohydrate, and are rich in folic acid, vitamins A, C and E and lutein, an antioxidant believed to protect eye health .

Sowing the seeds

Seeds, including sunflower, sesame and pumpkin, make a great snack. They're rich in protein and Essential Fatty Acids, as well as vitamins B and E and minerals – especially magnesium. Their high EFA content means they promote hormonal balance, helping to prevent PMT.

Select sweet peppers

Peppers are rich in fibre and high in vitamin C, betacarotene and potassium. They also contain the plant pigments lutein and zeaxanthin, thought to protect against macular degeneration, the main cause of blindness in the elderly.

Tomato sauce

Having tomato-based sauces on pasta and other dishes can help to protect against cancer, skin damage from the sun, and maintain eye health. Tomatoes contain lycopene, an antioxidant shown to prevent prostate and other cancers by neutralising free radicals (substances produced by the body when dealing with exposure to pollutants, such as cigarette smoke and overexposure to sunlight and illness) and believed to cause cell damage.

Lycopene may also help to keep eyes healthy and functioning well. Cooking tomatoes releases lycopene from the tomato cell walls, making it easier for the body to absorb. Lycopene dissolves in fat, so eating cooked tomatoes in the form of purees or sauce, with a source of fat such as cheese or olive oil, helps with absorption. So pizza, preferably served with a mixed salad, can be a healthy meal.

Wonderful walnuts

Walnuts appear to undo some of the harmful effects of eating saturated fats. As well as being a good source of omega-3's, walnuts contain arginine, an amino acid, and antioxidants. Research shows they can reduce hardening of the arteries —atherosclerosis—caused by saturated fats. It's thought the arginine is used by the body to make nitric oxide, which is needed to maintain the flexibility and elasticity of the arteries. This means the arteries can expand when needed, for increased blood flow. But eating walnuts won't make up for a diet high in saturated fats! Aim at reducing saturated fats as well. To gain the most benefit, eat them raw.

Say 'yes' to yoghurt

Eating live bio-yoghurt provides 'good' bacteria to boost your immune system Known as probiotics, these bacteria also have anti-inflammatory properties, which help combat the symptoms of irritable bowel syndrome and inflammatory bowel disease. They appear to treat diarrhoea in children, as well as relieving the symptoms of lactose intolerance and possibly reducing the risk of co-rectal cancer. They also help to beat bad breath.

Make way for watercress

Watercress is rich in antioxidants, beta-carotene, vitamins B1, B6 C, E and K as well as iron, magnesium and zinc. A daily serving may cut your risk of getting cancer by reducing damage to white blood cells and boosting their ability to resist damage by free radicals. It's also thought to be good for thyroid function.

Healing herbs

Many of us keep herbs in our food cupboard to add flavour and interest to meals, but did you know that studies confirm that ancient claims regarding their health-giving and medicinal properties are more than just folklore?

Many herbs contain even higher concentrations of antioxidants than fruit and vegetables and have anti-bacterial properties. They also contain phytochemicals and vitamins. Whilst we tend to consume herbs in small amounts, they nevertheless offer a tasty way to improve health.

Fresh herbs contain the most beneficial compounds, but if unavailable, dried herbs are still a valuable addition to your diet. They can be added to dishes as a healthy alternative to salt, and to enhance flavour. Some herbs make pleasant-tasting infusions. Use 30g (2tsp) of fresh herbs, or 15g (1tsp) of dried herbs per cup of boiling water. Simply pour the boiling water over the herb, cover and leave to stand for 5 to 10 minutes. Strain and add honey to taste. Drink whilst hot.

Growing your own herbs is easy. You can buy growing herbs from the fruit and vegetable section at your supermarket quite cheaply. Simply re-pot and place on a windowsill, or patio. Water and feed regularly.

Basil booster

Basil contains flavanoids including orientin and vicenin, which have been shown to protect cells from radiation and are antioxidant. Basil also contains volatile oils with antibacterial properties, helping to prevent some of the tummy bugs that cause diarrhoea. Another volatile oil in Basil, eugenol, has anti-inflammatory properties similar to those found in aspirin, making it beneficial to those with arthritis and other inflammatory conditions. Basil is believed to beat depression and ease cold symptoms too. It adds flavour to pastas and vegetable juices.

Quick tip

KEEP FLU AT BAY

Bay leaves contain traces of iron and phosphorous. They promote digestion and ease indigestion. They can ease flu symptoms by promoting sweating, when drunk as an infusion. The leaves are versatile, adding depth to savoury dishes, such as soups, stew and casseroles and enhancing the flavour of rice pudding.

Coriander cure

Coriander appears to ease indigestion, bloating and diarrhoea. Coriander seeds have a laxative effect. When crushed they can soothe mouth ulcers. Coriander also stimulates the appetite and helps to control the blood sugar. Research suggests it may help prevent colon cancer.

Colic relief

Dill soothes colic, easing gripe pains and dispersing flatulence. It's a common ingredient in commercial gripe waters, but you can make your own by adding one teaspoon (5g) of dill seeds to half a pint (500ml) of boiling water. Allow to cool and then strain. It's also antibacterial and is a diuretic.

Fen-tastic

In a two-month trial, fennel reduced period pain in young women. It's may also stimulate milk production in lactating mothers. Both the plant and seeds help relieve indigestion and flatulence. It's also a diuretic. A tea made from the crushed seeds is recommended for relief from cystitis and kidney stones. Fennel tea also eases coughs, bronchitis and blocked sinuses. Fennel can be eaten raw and finely sliced, in salads, or roasted in olive oil as a tasty accompaniment to chicken. It's best to remove the tough outer layer first. It isn't recommended for anyone at risk of seizures.

Lemon balm calm

Melissa officianalis, more commonly known as lemon balm, due to its nettle-like lemon-scented leaves, has long been used as a mood enhancer, because of its soothing and calming properties. It's said to ease tension and headaches, as well as reduce hyperactivity. It's also believed to boost memory by making brain cells more receptive to acetylcholene, a brain chemical linked to memory. The leaves can be chopped and added to fish or meat dishes, as well as drunk as a refreshing infusion. Or blend them into a pear smoothie to enhance the flavour.

Anti-ageing oregano

Also known as marjoram, weight for weight, oregano contains up to 20 times more antioxidants than other herbs, and up to four times more than blueberries.

When drunk as an infusion it's thought to relieve cold and flu symptoms. The oregano herb is safe to use during pregnancy, but oregano volatile oil isn't, as it may harm the baby.

Pick parsley for PMT

Parsley's diuretic properties relieve the water retention associated with periods. It may also normalise menstrual flow and relieve cramps and PMT. Taken daily, it can ease menopausal symptoms. It contains iron to help prevent anaemia. Other minerals such as calcium, magnesium and potassium are a general tonic. It's also a source of Vitamin C. Drinking a parsley infusion helps relieve cystitis. Chewing parsley freshens the breath. Other suggested uses are as a poultice for acne, eczema, bites, stings and sore eyes. It goes well with fish, or vegetable dishes or juices.

Peppermint pep-up

Peppermint stimulates the mind and clears headaches. It's very effective as a digestive aid, easing indigestion and flatulence and is good for IBS. When drunk as an infusion, it relieves cold and flu symptoms, clearing blocked nasal passages and promoting sweating. It may also protect against cancer. It can be added to salad dressings, savoury sauces and even desserts. In hot weather, blend mint leaves into your smoothies, to make them more refreshing and cooling.

Rosemary relief

7g—just over a teaspoon—of rosemary contains as many antioxidants as 55g of blueberries. It has antiseptic properties and stimulates digestion. It also freshens the breath. For a headache cure, or relief from cold symptoms, drink an infusion made from the leaves.

Wise up to sage

Sage is recommended as a memory enhancer and may also help prevent Alzheimer's. Research suggests the herb inhibits enzymes which attack acetycholene, a chemical implicated in learning and memory. It's also recommended for women suffering from hot flushes, both during and after the menopause. It's may reduce flushing by regulating hypothalamus function. It can be added to stews and casseroles, or drunk as a tea. It's not recommended for breastfeeding women, as it may reduce milk flow.

Tarragon tranquility

Tarragon has calming, sedative properties and tarragon tea is said to promote sleep. An appetite stimulant, it aids digestion. It can promote or increase menstrual flow, so should be avoided in pregnancy. It's commonly added to fish dishes.

Take thyme

Thyme is antibacterial and when drunk as an infusion can relieve cystitis, ease chest congestion and treat chronic coughs. It's also good for digestion and stimulates the circulation.

Spice of life

Spices are usually extracted from the bark, stem, and seeds of plants. They not only add flavour to your food, but also offer a variety of health benefits when consumed regularly. Even a pinch is enough to make a difference because of the potent chemicals spices contain, such as isothiocyanates, natural compounds which seem to inhibit cancers.

A pinch of black pepper

Black pepper stimulates the taste buds, which promote the secretion of hydrochloric acid in the stomach, improving digestion. It's reported to boost circulation and is antibacterial. It helps prevent water retention by promoting sweating and having a diuretic effect. It may help your body break down fat cells.

Clot buster

Researchers in India recently reported that cardamom has anti-blood-clotting properties, which means it could reduce the risk of heart attack and stroke.

Cardamom seeds also ease flatulence, colic and indigestion.

Cayenne soother

Cayenne is a hot, fiery spice made from ground chilli pods and seeds. It offers many of the benefits of chillis, such as relieving pain, boosting the circulation, and reducing blood clotting. Despite its fieriness, like chillis, it's reputed to soothe stomach ulcers and case indigestion.

A sprinkle of cinnamon

Sprinkling cinnamon on food and drinks can help prevent serious disease, as well as treat minor complaints. It stimulates the circulation, helping to reduce blood stickiness, which can cause clots, strokes and heart attacks. It's also good for the digestion, relieving nausea, flatulence and diarrhoea. The smell of cinnamon stimulates brain activity.

A compound in this spice helps your body convert glucose into energy more easily, helping to steady blood sugar levels. Studies suggest it may help prevent and treat type 2 Diabetes. It's also thought to reduce cholesterol and triglyceride levels. Cinnamon may boost metabolism and ease joint stiffness and pain too.

It tastes great sprinkled on a cappuccino or latte. Try it sprinkled on toast, porridge, or sweet potato. It adds flavour to apple crumble and baked apples.

Seek fenugreek

Fenugreek settles indigestion and soothes allergies. It contains saponins, natural detergents believed to lower cholesterol and triglyceride levels in the blood. Studies show fenugreek helps to control blood sugar in people with both type 1 and 2 diabetes. Historically it's been used to treat bronchitis and arthritis, wounds and absesses. In Chinese medicine, it's used to treat kidney problems.

Fenugreek can stimulate the uterus, so it's not advised during pregnancy, in case of miscarriage. Evidence suggests it may stop, or slow the growth of breast cancer.

"Once you have a spice in your home, you have it forever. Women never throw out spices."

Emma Bombeck

Calming cloves

Cloves contain various nutrients including Vitamin C, calcium and omega 3 oils. They're thought to soothe the stomach and ease nausea and vomiting. They also have a sedative effect and contain eugenol, which is antiseptic and anti-inflammatory relieving toothache, rheumatism and arthritis. They're traditionally used to treat respiratory conditions such as bronchitis and asthma. Cloves add flavour to vegetable and fruit dishes, as well as soups, curries and mulled wine.

Make room for cumin

Cumin seeds promote digestion and relieve flatulence, colic and diarrhoea. They may also prevent muscle cramps, reduce morning sickness and stimulate milk production.

Gain from garlic

Garlic contains sulphur compounds called diallyl sulphides and allicin, which are believed to fight viral and bacterial infections, boost immunity, prevent thrombosis, lower cholesterol and the risk of stomach and bowel cancers and protect against heart attacks and strokes. Leave chopped garlic for ten minutes to 'mature' before cooking, to help prevent the destruction of the beneficial compounds. Replace ordinary garlic bread with bread spread with crushed garlic and cooked in the oven until golden, for the health benefits of garlic, without the saturated fats.

To combat the smell of garlic on the breath, chew a sprig of parsley. Some chefs claim that you can avoid suffering from 'garlic-breath' by removing the yellow shoot in the middle of each bulb.

Ginger zinger

Chew raw ginger root to relieve nausea associated with stomach upsets, travel sickness, migraine and pregnancy. Though in the case of morning sickness, it's recommended that no more than one gram a day should be taken. To prevent travel sickness, eat ginger half an hour before your journey.

Ginger stimulates digestion and prevents indigestion, bloating and gas. It also soothes stomach ache and pain associated with diarrhoea and may reduce the risk of stomach ulcers.

It also blocks the effects of prostaglandins - substances which can cause inflammmation of blood vessels in the brain and lead to migraine. So it eases both the pain and nausea associated with migraine. Its anti-inflammatory properties also ease rheumatoid arthritis and menstrual cramps and may benefit osteoarthritis suffers as well.

To relieve menstrual pain, or cold and flu symptoms, sip hot ginger tea, made by pouring boiling water over three or four thin slices of ginger root and sweetened to taste, preferably with honey.

Anti-clotting properties, similar to those of aspirin, have been attributed to ginger. It boosts the circulation and lowers blood pressure and cholesterol, so it may help prevent heart attacks and strokes.

To benefit from ginger's health-giving properties and enjoy it's piquant flavour, use it in stir-fries, curries, cakes and biscuits.

Must-have mustard

Mustard seeds contain plant nutrients called glucosinolates and enzymes which break these down into isothiocyanates, which studies suggest prevent gastrointestinal and colorectal cancers. English mustard is made from brown and white mustard seeds.

By stimulating saliva production, mustard increases the appetite and aids digestion. It soothes upset stomachs, though too much can irritate. It's antiseptic, stimulates circulation and is a good source of minerals, particularly selenium, magnesium, iron and zinc.

Quick tip

NUTMEG FOR NAUSEA

Nutmeg is rumoured to ease nausea, flatulence and vomiting. It can also calm diarrhoea. It's claimed to clear up eczema, when applied as a paste made by mixing ground nutmeg with water. It's great in savoury dishes such as omelettes and cheese sauces, as well as desserts.

Paprika pick-me-up

Paprika is made from dried, red, mild to medium hot peppers. Like cayenne pepper, it contains capsaicin, and offers the same health benefits. It's sweeter and milder than cayenne.

Turmeric tonic

Turmeric is is the spice that gives curry powder its yellow colour. Its key health-boosting component is curcumin. Studies suggest this compound helps prevent Alzheimer's and joint inflammation and reduce cholesterol. It's also an anti-inflammatory and easing aches and pains and psoriasis. Evidence points to turmeric possibly having anti-cancer properties – particularly against bowel, colon and rectal cancers.

Vanilla chiller

Vanilla has a calming effect. Use vanilla pods or pure vanilla extract, rather than vanilla flavouring, to enhance the flavour of cakes and desserts.

Value vinegar

Studies show that adding vinegar to food helps you to feel full longer and therefore eat less.

Add a splash of ordinary malt, balsamic or white wine vinegar, or a vinaigrette dressing to dark leafy green vegetables – the acetic acid aids calcium absorption.

Vinegar seems to stabilise blood sugar levels by slowing down the absorption of glucose from food. It benefits those with type 2 diabetes by preventing the blood sugar from rising too high after a meal. Vinegar may help prevent the development of type 2 diabetes, though further research is needed to confirm this.

The three words
women most
want to hear
from a man are,
"You lost weight".

Lori Gottlieb

Healthy quenchers

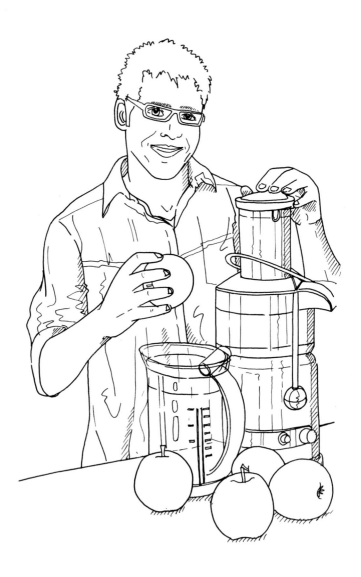

chapter 5
Healthy quenchers

Ensuring you drink adequate amounts of fluid is essential for good health. The body is around 70% water. We can go without food for around 5 weeks, but can only last about 5 days without fluids. Our cells, tissues, organs, and body processes all require water. You need around 6 to 8 225ml (8oz) glasses of liquid daily. But this can vary according to your age, gender, activity levels, and the temperature. Fruit and vegetables, with their high water content, will also hydrate you. Let your thirst guide you. Straw-coloured, odourless urine indicates you're getting enough fluids. Dark coloured, strong-smelling urine suggests you need to drink more water. Sugary drinks provide empty calories, and can lead to weight gain as well as tooth decay, so are best avoided. Some drinks can deliver particular health benefits, though in the case of tea, coffee, and alcohol, moderation is usually advised.

Water baby

Drinking between 1.5L and 2L of water each day is one of the easiest steps you can take to improve your health. Have a glass each morning, a glass between and with meals, and a glass at your bedside at night. Experts claim that being well-hydrated reduces the risk of obesity, constipation, kidney stones and urinary tract, and breast cancers, as well as preventing headaches and tiredness.

Ice is nice

Drinking water ice cold has been shown to boost the metabolism, because the body needs to heat it up before using it. Plain, still water is viewed as the healthiest choice. To make it even more refreshing, try adding a few sprigs of mint, or basil, or slices of cucumber, lime, or lemon.

MILK MAID

A recent study concluded that drinking 500ml (1pt) of milk daily more than halves the risk of insulin resistance, which can cause heart disease, stroke, and type 2 diabetes. Other research suggests that milk rehydrates the body after exercise for longer than expensive sports drinks, because it's removed from the body more slowly, due to the protein, fat, and sugar it contains.

Milk also contains vitamins and minerals, including calcium, and it doesn't cause tooth decay. Go for semi-skimmed or skimmed, as they contain less saturated fat than whole milk.

Just juicing

Juicing is another way of ensuring you benefit from fruit and vegetables. Enthusiasts claim that juicing releases the nutrients that are stored in the fibre of the whole fruit, so that they can be absorbed, rather than expelled with the fibre.

OPT FOR ORANGE JUICE

A glass of orange juice each day provides approximately 60ml of immunity-boosting vitamin C and folic acid, which helps prevent birth defects. If drunk with meals, it also increases iron absorption.

Smooth operator

Fruit smoothies are a great way to get your daily fruit quota. Because you're blending, rather than juicing, you get the benefits of the whole fruit, including the fibre.

This easy, energy-boosting recipe for 2, uses banana and natural yoghurt. Add any fruit you like.

1 large banana

2–3 handfuls of fruit

285ml/½ pint unsweetened natural yoghurt

Runny honey (optional)

Cinnamon, or nutmeg (optional)

Place the banana and your chosen fruit into a blender. Blend for 30 seconds. Add the natural yoghurt, and honey to taste. Blend again to a milk-shake consistency. Sprinkle with cinnamon or nutmeg and serve.

Stop for tea

Drinking tea—ordinary black, or green, or white oolong—provides an array of health benefits. Tea contains flavanoids, catechins and polyphenols – powerful antioxidants, believed to prevent heart disease and cancer. Green tea contains the most, followed by oolong and black teas. Tea also appears to promote normal blood pressure, by increasing the elasticity of arteries. But some research suggests that adding milk to tea blocks this effect.

Green tea is thought to assist weight loss by raising the metabolic rate. Evidence suggests that all three teas—including ordinary black tea—might also protect against stroke, osteoporosis, and bacterial and viral infections. Furthermore, your daily cuppa is anti-inflammatory and helps protect against allergies. Jigging the tea bag up and down a few times releases more of the beneficial antioxidants.

Despite recent claims to the contrary, it seems that tea is hydrating, provided you drink no more than six cups of average strength daily. This would give you a caffeine intake of around 300ml which shouldn't have a strong diuretic effect.

Tea helps you relax, because it contains a substance called theanine, which is believed to act as a tranquiliser, without affecting concentration. Recent tests showed that when tea drinkers are exposed to stress, their levels of the stress hormone cortisol drop much more quickly than those of non-tea drinkers.

Your dental health can benefit from drinking tea too. The fluoride it contains strengthens tooth enamel and also appears to prevent the growth of oral bacteria linked to bad breath and tooth decay.

Tea boosts insulin activity, helping to maintain a steady blood sugar, which helps to keep the appetite in check.

It's best to avoid drinking tea with a meal. Try to wait half an hour, because it contains tannins, which prevent your body from absorbing iron from non-meat sources, such as whole grains, peas or dried fruit. Tea also contains polyphenols which bind with iron, making absorption more difficult. Drinking your tea with a slice of lemon might help, because its vitamin C content aids iron absorption.

Redbush or Rooibos tea is lower in tannin than regular tea. It's also caffeine-free, so it's good to drink at bedtime, if caffeine tends to keep you awake.

HERBAL TEAS

Herbal teas make a refreshing alternative to tea and coffee, and provide the health-boosting properties of the herbs or spices they contain. Choose from a vast array, ranging from old favourites, ginger, peppermint and chamomile, to more exotic blends containing vanilla, or ginseng. Or make your own using fresh herbs – see chapter 4.

Coffee cure

Most people know that a cup of coffee can increase mental alertness and concentration, and counteract the effects of tiredness and fatigue. But did you know that coffee might have other health benefits?

A long-term study indicated that drinking three cups of coffee a day can reduce the risk of mental decline in old age and cut the risk of Alzheimer's by half. The elderly have higher levels of adenosine, a brain chemical that weakens gamma rhythms, which are involved in memory and learning processes. The caffeine in coffee appears to reduce the risk of memory loss and Alzheimer's by blocking the effects of adenosine.

Coffee might also reduce the risk of Parkinson's disease, gallstones and rectal cancer. A US study claimed that drinking four cups of coffee daily could reduce the incidence of gout in men.

Coffee can also help to relieve headaches, when drunk at the same time as taking painkillers such as ibuprofen. The caffeine content increases the painkilling effect, by improving absorption. A strong cup of coffee can help relieve migraines, which can occur when blood vessels in the head dilate. The caffeine constricts the blood vessels, relieving the painful symptoms of blood vessel dilation.

According to the Australian Institute of Sport, a cup of strong black coffee 1–2 hours before exercise stimulates the release of fats into the blood stream, which allows the body to burn fat as its main energy source, thus speeding up fat loss.

Another study suggests that drinking coffee and being active can inhibit skin cancer.

Coffee also seems to help stabilise blood sugar levels, reducing the storage of fat and the risk of type 2 diabetes.

Coffee quota

But, as always, moderation is the best policy. Drinking more than 4–5 cups of coffee daily might cause health problems. The caffeine in coffee is addictive and can cause anxiety, insomnia, tremors, and an irregular heartbeat. Women who drink 8 or more cups of coffee a day appear more likely to suffer a miscarriage or stillbirth. Heavy coffee drinkers also appear to be more at risk of heart disease, osteoporosis, and arthritis.

Quick tip

LOWER-CAL COFFEE

Be careful how you take your coffee. A large latte made with whole milk can contain around 18g (½oz) of saturated fat – nearly the recommended daily amount.

A cappuccino is slightly better, with around a third of the amount of saturated fat. Have it made with skimmed, or semi-skimmed milk, to reduce the saturated fat and calories. Or go for espresso. Avoid adding sugar and syrups, or topping with whipped cream, chocolate, or caramel. Cinnamon is a healthier choice.

Enjoy a tipple

A glass of red wine such as Pinot Noir, Cabernet Sauvignon, or Merlot, not only provides the benefits attributed to grapes, but also others linked with alcohol. These include increased HDL or 'good cholesterol', decreased fibrinogen—the body's blood clotting agent—and protection against Alzheimer's, colds and flu. Drinking white wine is also beneficial. All wine seems to improve lung health, but white has the most effect. It's thought that antioxidants in white wines mop up toxins in the blood and reduce inflammation.

But don't binge

Remember, moderation is the key! More than 3 units daily/ 14 units weekly for women and 4 units daily/21 units weekly for men, can have a detrimental effect on health. On average, one small glass of red wine contains 1.5 units of alcohol. A large glass typically contains 2 units.

Binge drinking, classified as drinking more than the recommended daily amount, appears to increase the risk of breast cancer in women, and stimulate tumour growth. It may also increase the risk of bowel cancer and is linked to cirrhosis of the liver. In can lead to obesity, because alcohol contains 7 calories per gram. Heavy drinking is also linked with high blood pressure, which increases the risk of strokes and heart attacks.

Pregnant women are advised not to drink alcohol. It crosses the placenta and enters the baby's bloodstream. It can damage developing organs and prevent normal growth and development. For all the latest advice on how to enjoy alcohol without damaging your health visit **www.drinkaware.co.uk**.

Sip slimline

Between 10% and 20% of your daily calorie intake might come from drinks. Sugar-sweetened beverages, sugary drinks, sweet alcoholic drinks and drinks with cream or full-fat milk are the main culprits. Try these changes – they're painless, and you could soon be slimmer and healthier:

- Cut your intake of sweet or creamy drinks by swapping short, fat glasses and mugs for tall thin glasses and mugs – you'll automatically drink less.

- Gradually reduce the amount of sugar you add, then cut it out altogether.

- Choose drinks made with semi-skimmed, or skimmed milk, instead of full-fat. Better still, drink tea and coffee without milk if you can.

- Swap sugary drinks such as coke and lemonade for sugar-free versions or, better still, water. A person who drinks 500ml (1pt) of coke or lemonade each day, would lose 11kg (25lbs) in weight each year simply by making this switch!

- Alternate drinking alcohol with low-calorie soft drinks, or water.

- Choose sugar free mixers such as diet coke.

- Drink wine spritzer, which is wine mixed with soda, instead of wine.

- Replace sugary alcopops with a shot of spirit and a low-calorie mixer.

- Swap a gin and tonic, containing 93 calories, for a gin and slimline tonic which contains only 53 calories.

Whenever I feel
like exercise,
I lie down until
the feeling passes.

Robert Hutchins

No time
for the gym?

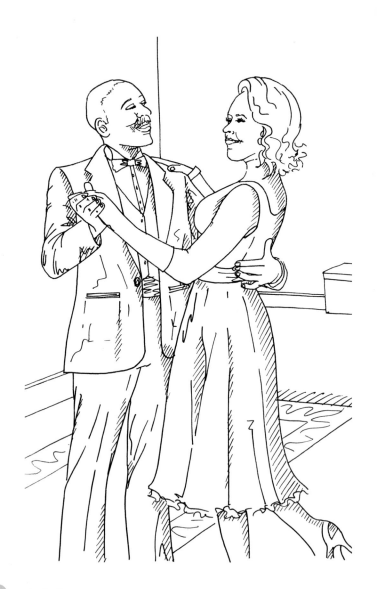

chapter 6
No time for the gym?

Physical activity helps you to lose weight by burning calories and boosting the metabolism. It can also reduce the risk of heart disease, type 2 diabetes, some cancers, osteoporosis, dementia, and Alzheimer's.

Apart from changes in diet, the other major factor in today's rapidly increasing obesity rates is the decrease in physical activity, due to the changes in lifestyles over the past few decades. Our parents and grandparents didn't go to the gym, but they were much slimmer and fitter, because their everyday lives involved far more activity.

A rise in car ownership and public transport means fewer people walk or cycle on a daily basis. Increased use of labour-saving domestic appliances and devices has reduced the amount of physical activity involved in running a home.

The current recommendations for adults are that they should take moderate intensity exercise, such as walking, for at least 30 minutes, for five or more days a week. For weight loss and management, aim at 60 minutes for at least five days a week. If you have an inactive lifestyle, it's best to build up gradually. For example, begin by walking ten minutes three times daily, before increasing to two fifteen minute and then one thirty minute walk daily.

Research suggests the best way to achieve fitness is by incorporating physical activity into your daily routine, just as our forebears did, rather than joining the gym; around £200 million is wasted on unused gym memberships each year, with people citing lack of time and boredom as the main reasons for their non-attendance.

Little and often

Being active several times a day benefits your metabolism more than doing one long bout of exercise. This is because during physical activity your metabolic rate increases and doesn't return to normal for up to two hours – depending on the intensity.

Make a stand

If you stand, rather than sit, you'll burn an extra 70 calories an hour. If you stood for 20 minutes a day, six days a week, you'd burn off 2lbs of fat in a year!

Leg it

Fit more walking into your daily routine. Walking is an aerobic exercise which increases cardiovascular fitness and lowers blood pressure, cholesterol and body fat, thus reducing the risk of strokes and heart attacks. Research reveals that whereas high intensity activity, such as a gym workout, tends to burn more carbohydrate than fat, moderate intensity exercise, like walking, burns more fat than carbohydrate. Other benefits include improved mental health, reduced risk of type 2 diabetes, breast and colon cancers and stronger bones and muscles. Park your car further from the office, or the shops. Get off the bus or train one stop earlier.

Walk away weight

Walking also aids weight control. Research shows that women take on average 5,000 steps daily and men 6,000. Overweight people take on average 1,500 to 2,000 fewer steps daily than those within a healthy weight range. So if you need to lose weight, try walking an extra 2,000 steps a day—roughly the equivalent of fifteen minutes of walking—and you'll burn around 450 calories a week. Even if you made no other changes in your lifestyle, in a year you would burn off around 6lbs in weight. Gradually increase your walking pace. The faster you walk, the more steps you'll clock up. 7,000 steps daily have been shown to improve fitness, but 10,000 can increase fitness dramatically and result in faster weight loss. Pedometers are cheap to buy and useful to determine whether you need to fit more walking into your daily routine.

Quick tip

WALKIES!

A recent survey indicated that dog owners take more exercise and are fitter than gym members. On average a dog walker clocks up 676 miles each year compared to only 468 miles for a gym-goer. Dog walkers have slightly lower blood pressure and their heart rates return to their resting rate more quickly than gym users. The average resting heart rate of dog walkers is lower than that of gym users. Dog owners generally take more exercise because they have to exercise their pets 'come rain or shine'. So, if you want to enjoy the benefits of your own canine personal fitness trainer, buy a dog, or offer to walk a neighbour's!

Be a domestic god/goddess

Household chores like vacuuming, dusting and cleaning, tone arm and leg muscles and increase the heart rate, making housework a good all-round cardiovascular exercise. Mopping, dusting, cleaning and vacuuming burns around 250 calories per hour, so it helps you control your weight. Work to the beat of your favourite CD and make cleaning more fun! Ironing burns around 140 calories per hour. Research shows if you approach housework as if you're doing a gym workout, you're more likely to lose weight! As you get fitter, you can speed up your domestic routine to burn off more calories.

Clean your own windows!

Clean your own windows to save money and give your body a workout. Climbing the ladders tones the leg muscles, whilst wiping firms the upper arms.

Peg it

Peg out clothes on the washing line intead of tumble-drying and it's not just the environment and your energy bills that'll benefit. As you reach up, your whole body gets a good stretch and carrying a full laundry basket outdoors works your arm muscles.

Quick tip

DITCH THE REMOTE
Throwing away the remote control will help you burn off around 1kg (2lbs) in weight in a year.

Walkie-talkie

Use a cordless or mobile phone and walk around the house as you talk.

Take TV breaks

Rather than sitting in front of the TV all evening, get up and walk around during the ad breaks, or in between programmes. You could even fit in a chore, like emptying the rubbish, or washing dishes. In three hours of viewing, you could clock up as much as forty five minutes of activity!

Go green-fingered

30 minutes of gardening offers the same benefits as a workout, especially if it includes digging. Even light gardening tasks can improve strength and agility.

General garden chores such as weeding, mowing and digging burn between 200 and 500 calories per hour and strengthen and tone muscles. Use a manual mower rather than an electrical one. Use a watering can, rather than a garden hose, to give your arm muscles a workout.

Gardening is also a weight-bearing exercise deemed more effective than jogging for strengthening bones. Sunlight on the skin stimulates the production of vitamin D, which helps the body to absorb bone-strengthening calcium, making gardening excellent protection against osteoporosis.

Wash the car by hand

Wash the car by hand, instead of going to the car wash.

> "If it weren't for the fact that the TV and the fridge were so far apart, some of us wouldn't get any exercise at all.

Joey Adams

Leave the car

For short trips, such as popping to the corner shop, leave the car at home and walk.

Stop the school run

If your children's school is within walking distance ditch the school run and walk them to school instead.

Family fitness

Too busy looking after your children to exercise? Pushing a pram or buggy around the park is good exercise for you and provides fresh air and a change of scenery for baby. Play ball games with older children. Take them for a long walk, or visit the local swimming baths.

Pace the platform

If your train is late, walk up and down the platform, rather than standing still. You can do the same at the bus stop.

Supermarket shape-up

Use a basket, rather than a trolley, when you only need a few groceries and you'll tone your shoulder and arm muscles.

Leave the lift

Taking the stairs instead of the lift will work your cardiovascular system, increase your level of fitness, tone your leg and thigh muscles and burn calories. If you drive, park your car at the top of the multistorey car park and use the stairs.

Be a disco diva

Dancing is an enjoyable way to get fit that can be combined with a healthy social life. It offers emotional, physical and mental health benefits, including increased cardiovascular fitness, stronger bones and muscles, improved co-ordination, agility and flexibility, improved balance and spatial awareness. One hour on the dance floor enables the average person to burn off 200 calories upwards – depending on the type of dancing. Strutting your stuff also improves your mental well-being, wards off dementia and develops social skills.

Get active at the office

Leave your desk and walk around regularly. Just a couple of minutes of activity every hour will equal one and a quarter hours of activity each working week. Walk to your colleagues' desks to pass on information instead of emailing. Walk to the water dispenser every hour for a refill and boost your hydration and activity levels. Make trips to the kitchen to make drinks.

Desk-ercises to beat DVT

Sitting at a desk for long periods poses the same risk of deep vein thrombosis as air travel does. It's important not to sit still for periods of longer than an hour. The following exercises help.

- Clench your calf and thigh muscles several times each hour.
- With your legs stretched out in front of you, raise your feet and hold for 1 minute.
- Sit with your feet directly in line with your knees. Then raise your feet and hold for 1 minute.

Walk the escalator

Walking up and down escalators helps to tone the bottom and burn calories!

Laugh yourself lean

Research suggests that laughing each day for about fifteen minutes burns as much energy as walking for half an hour, gives muscles a workout and raises the heart rate. You could lose up to 5 lbs in weight a year. So if you want to improve your figure and fitness the easy way, dig out those comedy videos and joke books and get giggling!

Fidget away fat

Scientists at the Mayo Clinic in Minnesota found that one of the biggest factors affecting a person's weight is their level of Non-Exercise Activity Thermogenesis—NEAT—more commonly known as fidgeting! They found that slim people tend to fidget more than overweight people and as a result burn up to 350 calories a day more.

If you're not a fidget, try to become one! Change position more often when standing or sitting. Tap your feet when seated. Pace up and down whilst waiting for the kettle to boil.

Temperature control

Turn down the thermostat at home and at the office and your body will burn fat to keep warm. Experts believe you can burn up to 250 calories a day trying to maintain a comfortable body temperature.

To the mind
that is still, the
whole universe
surrenders.

Lao Tzu

Stress busters

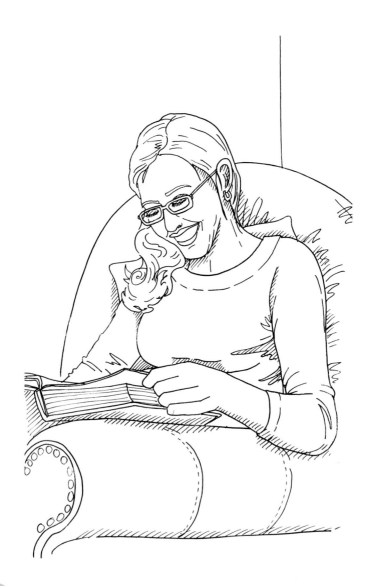

chapter 7
Stress busters

Stress is how our mind and body react to pressure, leaving us feeling inadequate or unable to cope. It depends on our perception of a situation and our ability to cope. What one person finds stressful, another might not.

The brain responds to stress by preparing our body to either stay and face up to the perceived threat, or to run away. This involves the release of hormones including adrenaline, noradrenaline, and cortisol into the bloodstream. As a result the heart-rate and breathing patterns speed up and we might sweat. Glucose and fatty acid levels in the blood increase to give us the energy to deal with the threat. This is commonly known as the 'fight or flight' response. Studies suggest that, over a prolonged period, these chemical effects of stress can be detrimental to health, leading to an increased risk of high blood pressure, CHD, stroke, cancer, obesity, diabetes, depression, and even memory loss and fertility problems.

If the cause of stress is not removed or controlled, cortisol levels remain high. The body then adapts to this constant state of emergency by increasing the appetite for high-energy foods and keeping a store of fat around the waist, near the vital organs, where it can be quickly converted back into energy. This is the most dangerous place to store fat because it's linked to an increased risk of CHD, stroke, and diabetes. Finding ways of dealing with stress is clearly essential for a long and happy life.

Bad habits

As well as overeating, we often deal with stress by adopting other unhealthy habits, such as smoking, and drinking too much alcohol, the ill-effects of which we are all aware.

With many of us living our lives at an increasingly fast pace and often under pressure to achieve and perform, stress has become a major cause of ill-health. In the UK, each day an estimated 270,000 people take time off work due to stress-related illness, at a cost of over £10 billion.

Quick tip

KEEP A STRESS JOURNAL
For a couple of weeks keep a record of situations, times, places, and people that make you feel stressed. Once you've identified your stressors, find ways to avoid or minimise them.

Manage your time

If you constantly feel under pressure and stressed due to a lack of time you could look at how you use it. Keep a diary for a few days to see where your time goes and then see which activities you can cut out, or reduce, to make time for the things that are most important to you. If you commute, use the time positively, rather than just gazing out of the window. For example, read a book, plan your diary, or relax, listening to your favourite music.

JUST SAY 'NO'

If you feel overburdened with chores and your stress levels are rising as a result, try saying "no" to non-essential tasks you don't have time for or just don't want to do.

What a to do!

Make a 'To-Do' list to help prevent yourself from feeling overwhelmed by the tasks you need to do. Then prioritise, so that you do the most urgent jobs first. You'll feel more in control and organised. You won't forget to do something that has a deadline or is important. 'To Do' lists work well both at work and at home, helping you to be more efficient and less stressed.

Think positive

Affirmations are positive statements you make about and to yourself, which help raise your self esteem. The higher your self-esteem, the more able you will be to deal with life's challenges, and you'll be less likely to suffer from stress. Remember stress arises from your perception of a situation, rather than from the situation itself. If you find yourself in a situation which is causing you stress, visualise yourself coping with it and use an affirmation. For example, if you have a forthcoming job interview or exam that is worrying you, picture yourself performing well and use a positive affirmation such as "I am capable of doing this job" or "I can pass this exam". This should increase your confidence in your ability to deal with the situation, and as a result it should become less stressful.

Live in the present

Mindfulness has been shown to reduce stress levels. It has its roots in Buddhism and involves focusing on the here and now, rather than worrying about the past or future. It's based on the philosophy that we can't change the past, or predict the future, but we can affect what's happening right now. By living fully in the present you can perform to the best of your ability, whereas worrying about the past and future can hamper how you function now, and increase stress levels unnecessarily.

CLEAR CLUTTER
Getting rid of unused items and tidying your home, or work space, helps you to feel in control, and this in turn leads to you feeling calmer.

Laugh a lot

Laughter really is the best medicine! Not only does it make you fitter, it also relieves stress and boosts the immune system. After a bout of laughter, the levels of cortisol and other stress hormones in the body reduce. A good belly-laugh also relaxes the muscles in the upper body.

Pet therapy

Stroking your pet dog or cat lowers your blood pressure and reduces stress. Research indicates that the heart rate slows down and the body stops producing the stress hormones cortisol and adrenaline.

The sound of music

Listen to your favourite CD. Evidence suggests that taking time out to listen to music you enjoy reduces anxiety and might even relieve pain.

Chew gum

Chewing gum seems to reduce muscular tension and the effects of stress on the brain. It appears to stimulate parts of the brain with a role in lowering tension and may reduce the production of stress hormones.

Go back to nature

Go back to nature to reduce your stress levels. Activities such as looking at the sea, going for a walk in the park or the countryside, or even gardening, have proven to reduce heart rate, blood pressure and muscle tension. Experts think that the higher levels of negative ions near areas with running water, trees and mountains may be partly responsible. Others link it to 'biophilia' – the idea that man has a natural affinity with nature. Research suggests people living near green areas enjoy a longer lifespan and better health, than those who live in urban environments.

Walk away worries

Walking reduces stress by stimulating the production of endorphins – natural tranquilizers which give a feeling of well-being, reduce depression, anxiety and stress. As a result walkers feel more positive and able to deal with problems, which leads to further reductions in stress levels.

Sunshine soother

Exposure to natural sunlight raises serotonin levels in the brain, boosting both mood and the ability to deal with stress. But make sure that you follow current advice regarding sunshine exposure:

- Stay in the shade from 11am-3pm.
- Ensure you never burn.
- Cover up.
- Take extra care with children.
- Use factor 15+ sunscreen.

Social support

Research shows that people who have a good social network tend to enjoy better mental health than those who don't. So make time to see family and friends regularly.

Wind down at work …

Whilst too many interruptions in the form of emails, text messages, phone calls and colleagues chatting can cause the work to pile up and stress levels to rise, being sociable at work is a stress reducer. A chat with colleagues over a cuppa, and encouragement and support from your supervisor all help to keep you happy at work.

Plant power

Placing a plant on your desk can reduce your stress levels. Researchers believe they reduce pollutant levels in the air and improve humidity. Also nature has a calming effect on people.

SWITCH OFF !

To help you switch off, switch off your mobile phone or Blackberry outside of work and especially on holiday!

Take a break

Try to schedule regular 'me-time' breaks into you daily routine. Even 2 x 15-minute breaks during your working day, during which you do whatever you want, can help to reduce feelings of stress. Something as simple as having a cup of tea and a chat, or reading the newspaper, can have a positive effect as it can take your mind off your work situation.

Breathe deep

Deep breathing has been shown to reduce the heart rate, relax muscles and release tension. Next time you feel stressed, try this simple exercise. Inhale slowly to a count of 5, allowing your tummy to expand, hold for a count of 5 and then breathe out slowly to a count of 5, whilst slowly flattening your tummy. Repeat up to 10 times.

Two-minute revitaliser

Every 2 or 3 hours try this 2-minute exercise to release tension and revive energy. Slowly massage your temples, gently but firmly, for 1 minute in an anti-clockwise direction and then for 1 minute clockwise. At the same time picture a relaxing scene, e.g. lying on the beach on holiday or relaxing in front of a big log fire – whatever conjures up relaxation for you.

LIGHT A CANDLE
A lit candle has a calming, almost hypnotic effect.
Focussing on a lit candle whilst practising deep breathing
is a simple form of meditation.

Sniff lavender

Japanese researchers found that sniffing lavender oil for
5 minutes a day dramatically reduces the stress hormone
cortisol. Rosemary oil was found to be equally effective.

Touch therapy

Massage is one of the oldest and most effective methods
of counteracting stress. Daily tensions and stress can make
us uptight and lead to pain and muscle stiffness. The Greek
philosopher Hippocrates, the 'father of medicine', recognised
the value of massage, claiming it "can loosen a joint that is
too rigid". Massage involves touch – a powerful tool that can
ease away tensions, aches and pains. It works by stimulating
the release of endorphins—the body's own painkillers—and
serotonin, a brain chemical associated with relaxation.
It also decreases the level of stress hormones in the blood
and improves blood circulation.

Make your own massage oil by mixing a few drops of your
favourite aromatherapy oil, e.g. lavender, chamomile or ylang
ylang, into a carrier oil such as almond or grapeseed. The
easiest way to enjoy the benefits of massage is for you and
your partner to massage each other's back, neck, and shoulders

using the basic techniques listed below:

Stroking/**effleurage** – glide both hands over the skin in rhythmic fanning or circular motions.

Kneading – using alternate hands, squeeze and release flesh between fingers and thumbs, as if you're kneading dough.

Friction – use your thumbs to apply even pressure to static points, or make small circles, on either side of the spine.

Hacking – relax your hands and use the sides quickly and alternately to give short, sharp taps all over.

Playing some relaxing music at the same time can enhance the feeling of relaxation.

Hand-y relaxer

Next time you're feeling stressed and tense, use your thumbs to apply pressure to each of your solar plexus reflexes, which are in the middle of each palm, about two-thirds of the way up.

Meditate

Learn Transcendental Meditation – it's a simple technique which, if practised daily, has been shown to relieve stress and tiredness, and increase energy and the ability to think clearly. To learn more go to www.t-m.org.uk.

Useful web sites

www.stressbusting.co.uk – a website offering a stress test to enable you to discover your 'stress quotient' and lots more tips to help you deal with stress.

Oh sleep!
   it is a gentle thing,
Beloved from
   pole to pole!

Samuel Taylor Coleridge

Sleep tight

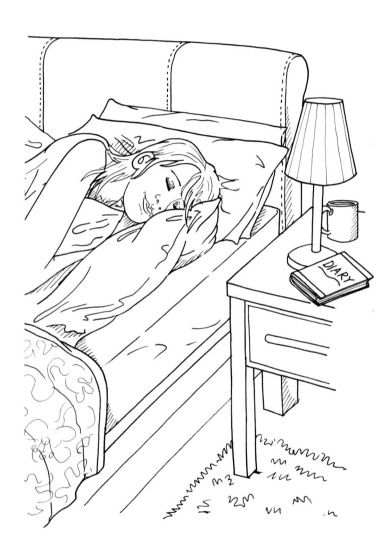

chapter 8
Sleep tight

Getting the right amount of good-quality sleep is vital for good health. Studies show that sleeping less than five hours a night increases the risk of heart disease, stroke, diabetes, obesity, depression, and decreases immunity. The increased risk of heart disease has been blamed on the link between too little sleep and higher levels of cortisol, the hormone linked with stress, in the bloodstream. The pre-disposition to diabetes in men might be due to reduced levels of testosterone noted among male poor sleepers. Testosterone appears to help prevent diabetes. Sleep deprivation can affect hormones which control appetite – see the chapter on eating less. Insomnia can also lead to inefficiency and more time off work.

Lack of sleep can affect mood and lead to relationship problems. It can also affect co-ordination, reaction time and judgement and increase risk-taking behaviour, leading to a greater possibility of involvement in road or other accidents. Evidence suggests that overall, people who sleep less than six hours a night don't live as long as those who sleep seven to eight hours. Paradoxically, sleeping longer than this might also shorten the lifespan. If you sleep an average of seven to eight hours nightly and generally feel alert, you're probably getting enough sleep.

The wake/sleep cycle is governed by the circadian rhythm and the sleep homeostat. The circadian rhythm is like an internal clock, which determines when we feel like sleeping and waking. Exposure to natural light and darkness, meal times and exercise patterns can all affect it. The sleep homeostat is a mechanism controlled by brain chemicals, such as melatonin, that ensures you get enough sleep.

If you have problems falling asleep, wake often during the night, or early in the morning, try some of these lifestyle changes to help you rebalance your wake/sleep cycle.

Make your bedroom a peaceful haven

Ensure your bed is comfortable and inviting, with fresh bedding. Replace the mattress if necessary. Buy the biggest bed you can afford, so that you or your partner can escape if one of you has a restless night. Make sure curtains and blinds keep the room dark – light interferes with the production of the sleep hormone melatonin. Line your curtains with blackout cloth, or invest in some blackout blinds.

Quick tip

SLEEP STEALERS

Don't have a TV in the bedroom, as watching TV last thing at night can overstimulate the brain and make it harder to switch off. Avoid using a computer late at night, as it can have a similar effect. The bright lights on TV and computer screens might also interfere with the hormones that regulate the wake/sleep cycle.

Keep your cool

Your brain tries to reduce your body temperature at night to slow down your metabolism. So to encourage sleep keep your room fairly cool – around 16°C (60°F) and keep it airy. Cotton nightwear and bedding are best for helping you to maintain a steady temperature, because cotton absorbs sweat.

If hot flushes wake you at night, sleep with a cotton sheet under the duvet. When a flush strikes, you can throw off the duvet and still have a light cover.

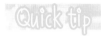

GET OUT MORE!

Research suggests that spending time outdoors during the day helps you sleep better at night. Exposure to sunlight stops the production of melatonin, making it easier for your body to produce the hormone at night, helping you to fall asleep more easily and sleep more soundly.

Enjoy exercise

Taking exercise late afternoon or early evening will increase your body temperature and metabolism, both of which will drop after about 5 hours, making you feel drowsy and ready to sleep. Also, research shows that people who exercise for at least half an hour 4 times a week sleep around 40 minutes longer than those who don't. Too little exercise can cause restlessness and problems with sleeping.

Coffee curfew

Coffee contains caffeine, which acts as a stimulant. The effects can last for hours, so try not to drink coffee after 2pm. The same goes for cola. Whilst tea generally contains less than half as much caffeine—around 50mg—it's advisable not to overdo it near bed time if you have trouble dropping off. Alternatively, try Redbush or Rooibos tea, which is caffeine-free.

Avoid alcohol …

If you have trouble sleeping, avoid drinking alcohol near bedtime. Alcohol in general has a relaxing effect, helping you to fall asleep, but it is a stimulant making you more likely to wake up during the night. It's also a diuretic, so you're more likely to wake up to make trips to the loo.

… but sip Sauvignon

Whilst alcohol in general is not recommended at bedtime – a glass of Cabernet Sauvignon, Merlot, or Chianti is. These wines contain grape skins that are rich in the sleep hormone melatonin.

Quick tip

LIMIT LIQUIDS
Generally avoid drinking large quantities of any liquid near bedtime to avoid waking to make trips to the bathroom.

No nicotine

As well as being extremely damaging to your health in general, nicotine is a stimulant, so if you must smoke, avoid smoking at bedtime. If you're using nicotine patches to help you stop smoking, be warned that they might cause vivid nightmares!

DON'T STUFF OR STARVE
Try not to overeat near bedtime, as it might cause you discomfort and prevent you from sleeping soundly. Likewise, don't eat too little, as hunger pangs could keep you awake, or wake you during the night.

Foods to help you snooze …

Bananas are suitable for bedtime snacking because they are rich in tryptophan, the precursor to serotonin. Other foods rich in tryptophan include chicken, turkey, dairy foods, eggs, beans, rice, oats, nuts, seeds, dates, and whole grains. A carbohydrate-rich meal increases the brain's uptake of tryptophan.

Magnesium-rich foods such as seafoods, nuts, seeds, whole grains and cooked green vegetables help to relax muscles and avoid night cramps. So an evening meal containing brown rice or pasta with chicken, or turkey and a green vegetable would help ensure a good night's sleep. A bedtime snack of nuts or seeds would also be beneficial.

… and the ones to avoid

If you have trouble dropping off, try to avoid foods which contain tyramine, an amino acid which stimulates the production of adrenaline. These include the nightshade family of vegetables, i.e. potatoes, tomatoes, courgettes, aubergines and spinach. Tyramine is also found in aged or fermented foods such as beers, tinned meats, mature cheeses, salami, pepperoni, and yeast extract .

Lettuce sleep

Lettuce has been recommended as a bed-time snack since Roman times. It has a sedative effect, because it contains a substance called lactucarium, which has a similar effect as opium. Try adding it to a chicken or turkey sandwich.

Chilli out

Include chilli in your evening meal! Chillis contain capsaicin, which appears to help regulate the sleep cycle, allowing you to fall asleep more easily and wake up feeling more refreshed.

Quick tip

WRITE AWAY YOUR WORRIES
Studies suggest that stress and anxiety can disrupt sleep. If anxiety prevents you from sleeping, try writing a list of the things you need to do, or issues that are worrying you and possible solutions, before bedtime, so that you don't mull things over when you should be sleeping.

Dim the lights

Ease your body into sleep mode by reducing the level of light in the evening. This will encourage the production of the sleep hormone melatonin. A dimmer switch is ideal for this, or try winding down in lamp or candlelight.

Bedtime ritual

Try to stick to a routine at bedtime. Follow the same ritual in the same order – for example you might take a bath first, followed by a milky drink and then read for 10 minutes to help you wind down, before reaching for the bedside lamp. Try going to bed at the same time each night. Your brain should eventually become programmed to enable you to fall asleep as a response to following the same regular steps.

Take to the tub

Take a warm bath before bed. The heat relaxes the muscles and mind. Also, sleep is normally preceded by a slight drop in body temperature which gives your body the 'message' that it's time for sleep. A warm bath raises your temperature slightly and the subsequent drop in temperature is conducive to sleep.

Enjoy a milky nightcap

A hot milky drink makes an ideal nightcap. Milk not only contains tryptophan, from which the brain produces serotonin, a hormone that makes you sleepy, it also contains calcium, which aids the process and helps you to relax. Add a vanilla pod and a little honey, for a delicious and calming bedtime drink.

Calming chamomile

Drinking chamomile tea is a well-known antidote to insomnia. It contains the amino acid glycine, which is a muscular and nerve relaxant. If you dislike the taste try adding 2 or 3 bags to a hot bath to enjoy the benefits without having to drink it!

Quick tip

SLEEP EASY WITH ESSENTIAL OILS

Various essential oils have calming, sedative properties. Most notably lavender, chamomile, valerian, neroli, and rose. Add them to the bath, sprinkle them on your pillow, or mix with a carrier oil such as almond, for a bedtime massage. If a stuffy nose due to cold or flu causes sleeping problems, sprinkle a few drops of eucalyptus or tea tree oil on your pillow.

Breathe deep

Try deep abdominal breathing to help you relax at bedtime. Aim to inhale slowly through your nostrils to a count of 3 whilst expanding your stomach. Hold for a count of 3 and then exhale through your mouth, counting to 6 whilst flattening your stomach. Repeat 5 times.

Sleep regulator

To help regulate your sleep/wake cycle try a spot of DIY reflexology to stimulate your pineal gland. Using your thumb and fore-finger, massage the fleshy part about two-thirds of the way up your big toes, for 1 or 2 minutes before bedtime.

DON'T CLOCKWATCH!

If you wake during the night, try not to look at the clock as you might start worrying about how long you have left to sleep which might prevent you from dropping off again. Instead, keep your eyes shut and try deep breathing to ease yourself back to sleep.

Sleep Council

For more advice on how to get a good night's sleep, including how to choose a new bed or mattress, and details of a helpline providing support for insomnia sufferers, visit **www.sleepcouncil.com**.

Index

'The Greatest Tips in the World' books

Baby & Toddler Tips
by Vicky Burford
ISBN 978-1-905151-70-7

Barbeque Tips
by Raymond van Rijk
ISBN 978-1-905151-68-4

Cat Tips by Joe Inglis
ISBN 978-1-905151-66-0

Cookery Tips
by Peter Osborne
ISBN 978-1-905151-64-6

Cricketing Tips
by R. Rotherham & G. Clifford
ISBN 978-1-905151-18-9

Dog Tips by Joe Inglis
ISBN 978-1-905151-67-7

Etiquette & Dining Tips
by Prof. R. Rotherham
ISBN 978-1-905151-21-9

Freelance Writing Tips
by Linda Jones
ISBN 978-1-905151-17-2

Gardening Tips
by Steve Brookes
ISBN 978-1-905151-60-8

Genealogy Tips
by M. Vincent-Northam
ISBN 978-1-905151-72-1

Golfing Tips
by John Cook
ISBN 978-1-905151-63-9

Horse & Pony Tips
by Joanne Bednall
ISBN 978-1-905151-19-6

Household Tips
by Vicky Burford
ISBN 978-1-905151-61-5

Personal Success Tips
by Brian Larcher
ISBN 978-1-905151-71-4

Podcasting Tips
by Malcolm Boyden
ISBN 978-1-905151-75-2

Property Developing Tips
by F. Morgan & P. Morgan
ISBN 978-1-905151-69-1

Retirement Tips
by Tony Rossiter
ISBN 978-1-905151-28-8

Sex Tips
by Julie Peasgood
ISBN 978-1-905151-74-5

Slimming & Healthy Living Tips
by Wendy Green
ISBN 978-1-905151-31-8

Travel Tips
by Simon Worsfold
ISBN 978-1-905151-73-8

Pet Recipe books

The Greatest Feline Feasts in the World by Joe Inglis
ISBN 978-1-905151-50-9

The Greatest Doggie Dinners in the World by Joe Inglis
ISBN 978-1-905151-51-6

'The Greatest in the World' DVDs

The Greatest in the World – Gardening Tips
presented by Steve Brookes

The Greatest in the World – Yoga Tips
presented by David Gellineau and David Robson

The Greatest in the World – Cat & Kitten Tips
presented by Joe Inglis

The Greatest in the World – Dog & Puppy Tips
presented by Joe Inglis

For more information about currently available
and forthcoming book and DVD titles please visit:

www.thegreatestintheworld.com

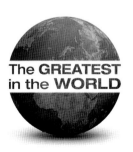

or write to:

The Greatest in the World Ltd
PO Box 3182
Stratford-upon-Avon
Warwickshire CV37 7XW
United Kingdom

Tel / Fax: +44(0)1789 299616
Email: info@thegreatestintheworld.com

The author

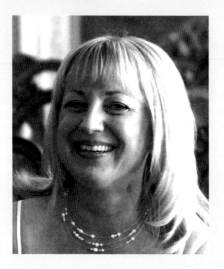

Wendy Green has been interested in health and weight control since her teens. In 2000 she gained a First Class Honours Degree in Health studies, which included the study of Psychology, Nutrition, Biology, The Sociology of Health, Complementary Therapies and Health Promotion. Since then, she's delivered seminars and lectures in Health Promotion and Nutrition, both in Further and Higher Education. She's currently working in the Voluntary Sector as a Co-ordinator and Trainer on 'Focus on Health', a health project delivering a health promotion programme to the deaf community.